CLINICAL GUIDE TO

BONE AND MINERAL METABOLISM IN CKD

EDITOR

KLAUS OLGAARD

CONTENTS

Contributors iv

Foreword vii
Garabed Eknoyan, Norbert Lameire, Sharon M. Moe, Tilman B. Drüeke

Preface ix
Klaus Olgaard

1. Mineral Homeostasis and Bone Physiology 3
William G. Goodman and L. Darryl Quarles

2. Pathophysiology and Clinical Manifestations of Renal Osteodystrophy 31
Arnold Felsenfeld and Justin Silver

3. Diagnosis of Bone and Mineral Disorders 45
Kevin J. Martin, Masafumi Fukagawa, and Hartmut H. Malluche

4. Morbidity and Mortality Associated with Abnormalities in
Bone and Mineral Metabolism in CKD 77
Geoffrey A. Block and John Cunningham

5. Vascular Calcification in CKD 93
Gérard M. London, Paulo Raggi, and Keith A. Hruska

6. Treatment Approaches in CKD 111
Tilman B. Drüeke, Sharon M. Moe and Craig B. Langman

7. Post-Transplant Bone Disease 141
Klaus Olgaard and Stuart M. Sprague

8. Renal Osteodystrophy in Children 155
Isidro B. Salusky and Otto Mehls

9. Osteoporosis and Hypogonadism in CKD Patients 175
José R. Weisinger and Mary B. Leonard

Appendix
Table 1. Conversion Factors: Metric Units to SI Units 191
Table 2. Classification of Chronic Kidney Disease (CKD) .192
Table 3. Target Levels for PTH, Calcium, and Phosphorus by Stage of CKD 193
Table 4. Calcium Content of Common Calcium-Based Phosphate Binders 194
Table 5. Summary of Clinically Useful Phosphate Binders 195
Table 6. Abbreviations and Acronyms 196

CONTRIBUTING AUTHORS

Geoffrey A. Block, MD
Director of Clinical Research
Denver Nephrologists, P.C.
Denver, CO, USA

John Cunningham, MD, FRCP
Professor of Nephrology
The Royal Free Hospital and University
College London
London, UNITED KINGDOM

Tilman B. Drüeke, MD, FRCP
Research Director and Associate Professor
Inserm Unit 507 and Div. of Nephrology
Necker Hospital
Université Paris 5
Paris, FRANCE

Arnold J. Felsenfeld, MD
Professor of Medicine
Departments of Medicine, West Los
Angeles VA Medical Center and UCLA
Los Angeles, CA, USA

Masafumi Fukagawa, MD, PhD, FJSIM,
FASN
Kobe University School of Medicine
Division of Nephrology & Dialysis
Kobe, JAPAN

William G. Goodman, MD
Professor of Medicine
David Geffen School of Medicine at UCLA
Division of Nephrology
UCLA Medical Center
Los Angeles, CA, USA

Keith A. Hruska, MD
Director Pediatric Nephrology
Professor of Pediatrics, Medicine and Cell
Biology
Washington University in St. Louis
Saint Louis, MO, USA

Craig B. Langman, MD
Isaac A. Abt, MD Professor of Kidney
Diseases
Feinberg School of Medicine, Northwestern
University
Head, Kidney Diseases
Children's Memorial Hospital
Chicago, IL, USA

Mary B. Leonard, MD, MSCE
Asst. Professor of Pediatrics and
Epidemiology
Children's Hospital of Philadelphia
Division of Nephrology
Center for Clinical Epidemiology and
Biostatistics
University of Pennsylvania School of Medicine
Philadelphia, PA, USA

Gérard M. London MD
Hemodialysis and Hypertension Department
Manhes Hospital
Fleury-Mérogis, FRANCE

Hartmut H. Malluche MD, FACP
Robert G. "Robin" Luke Chair in Nephrology
Professor and Chief
Division of Nephrology, Bone & Mineral
Metabolism
Department of Medicine
University of Kentucky, Chandler Medical
Center
Lexington, KY, USA

Kevin J. Martin, MB, BCh, FACP
Professor of Internal Medicine
Director, Division of Nephrology
Saint Louis University Health Sciences Ctr.
Saint Louis, MO, USA

Otto Mehls, MD
Professor of Pediatrics
University Children's Hospital
Heidelberg, GERMANY

Sharon M. Moe, MD, FACP, FAHA
Associate Professor of Medicine
Vice Chair for Research
Indiana University
Div of Nephrology, OPW 526
Indianapolis, IN, USA

Klaus Olgaard, MD
Professor of Medicine
University of Copenhagen,
Department of Nephrology P2132,
Rigshospitalet, DK-2100
Copenhagen, DENMARK

L. Darryl Quarles, MD
Summerfield Endowed Professor of
Nephrology
Vice Chair, Depart. of Internal Med.
Director, The Kidney Institute & Division of
Nephrology, MS 3018
University of Kansas Medical Center
Kansas City, KS, USA

Paolo Raggi, MD
Professor of Medicine
Tulane University School of Medicine
SL48/ Dept. of Med., Sect. of Cardiology
New Orleans, LA, USA

Isidro B. Salusky, MD
Professor of Pediatrics
Division of Pediatric Nephrology
Director, Pediatric Dialysis Program
Director, General Clinical Research Center
David Geffen School of Medicine at UCLA
Los Angeles, CA, USA

Justin Silver FRCP, PhD
Professor of Medicine
Chief, Nephrology and Hypertension
Services
Hadassah Hospital
Hadassah Hebrew University Medical Center
Jerusalem, ISRAEL

Stuart M. Sprague, DO
Chief, Division of Nephrology and
Hypertension
Evanston Northwestern Healthcare
Professor of Medicine
Feinberg School of Medicine
Northwestern University
Evanston, IL, USA

José R. Weisinger, MD, FACP
Professor of Medicine
Universidad Central de Venezuela
Head, Clinical Research Laboratory
Division of Nephrology
Hospital Universitario de Caracas
Caracas, VENEZUELA

CONTRIBUTING REVIEWERS

Gavin J. Becker, MD, FRACP
Department of Nephrology
Royal Melbourne Hospital
Victoria, AUSTRALIA

Ezequiel Bellorin-Font, MD
University Hospital of Caracas
Caracas, VENEZUELA

Kai-Uwe Eckardt, MD
Professor of Medicine
Chief, Nephrology/Hypertension Section
University Hospital of Erlangen
Erlangen, GERMANY

Garabed Eknoyan, MD
Baylor College of Medicine
Houston, TX, USA

Denis P. Fouque, MD, PhD
Department of Nephrology
Edouard Herriot Hospital
Lyon, FRANCE

Norbert H. Lameire, MD
Chief Renal Division
University Hospital Ghent
Nephrology Department
Ghent, BELGIUM

Adeera Levin, MD, FRCPC
Professor of Medicine
St. Paul's Hospital
Vancouver, BC, CANADA

Nathan W. Levin, MD, FACP
Renal Research Institute
New York, NY, USA

Jérôme Rossert, MD, PhD
Department of Nephrology
Tenon Hospital
AP-HP and Pierre and Marie Curie
University
Paris, FRANCE

Raymond Vanholder, MD
Chief Renal Division
University Hospital Ghent
Nephrology Department
University Hospital
Ghent, BELGIUM

Rowan Walker, MD, MBBS, FRACP
Department of Nephrology
Royal Melbourne Hospital
Victoria, AUSTRALIA

FOREWORD

Chronic kidney disease (CKD) is a worldwide public health problem of increasing prevalence and adverse outcomes, including progressive loss of kidney function, cardiovascular disease, and premature death. Strategies to improve the morbidity and mortality associated with CKD require an evidence-based global effort directed at the detection and management of the earlier stages of CKD.

The rationale for a global initiative is simple and self-evident. The epidemic of CKD is global. The adverse outcomes of CKD are universal, as are the underlying evidence-based strategies for the prevention, detection, evaluation, and treatment of CKD patients. Although risk factors and available resources for care vary regionally, it is important to increase the efficiency of utilizing available expertise and resources to develop a uniform and global public health approach to the worldwide epidemic of CKD, which can be adopted and adapted to address local needs. It is in an attempt to address these needs that the Kidney Disease: Improving Global Outcomes (KDIGO) initiative was launched in 2002.

KDIGO is an independently incorporated organization governed by an international Board of Directors with the stated mission to "improve the care and outcomes of kidney disease patients worldwide through promoting coordination, collaboration, and integration of initiatives to develop and implement clinical practice guidelines."

Information on the strategies and projects undertaken by KDIGO to elevate international awareness of the epidemic of kidney disease and provide a public health approach to CKD can be obtained at: www.kdigo.org. Amongst those is the Global Bone and Mineral Initiative (GBMI) established to address one of the common and serious complications of CKD.

The processes causing disordered bone and mineral metabolism have their onset in the early stages of CKD, persist throughout the course of progressive loss of kidney function, and are aggravated during replacement therapy following the onset of kidney failure. Apart from the musculoskeletal abnormalities, the long-term effects of these derangements on soft-tissue calcification account for much of the morbidity and mortality of these patients. Thus, the prevention of these disturbances and their appropriate management throughout the course of CKD are extremely important in improving the outcomes of CKD patients.

The present *Clinical Guide to Bone and Mineral Metabolism in CKD* represents one of the several projects adopted by GBMI in its multi-pronged approach to the problem of bone and mineral metabolism in CKD. The *Clinical Guide* has the specific educational mission of disseminating to the professional community the existing and newly acquired knowledge of the complex derangements in bone and mineral metabolism in CKD. On behalf of KDIGO and its GBMI, we would like to express our gratitude to all the authors for their valuable contributions to the *Clinical Guide*.

It is hoped that this first edition of the Clinical Guide will prove to be a quick reference and handy tool for the complex pathophysiological aspects of a rather intricate disease. Your suggestions and comments for improvement of future editions are welcome.

Garabed Eknoyan, MD
KDIGO Co-chair

Norbert Lameire, MD
KDIGO Co-chair

Sharon Moe, MD
GBMI Co-chair

Tilman Drüeke, MD
GBMI Co-chair

PREFACE

Over the last decade, there have been significant advances in the field of bone and mineral metabolism in patients with chronic kidney disease (CKD). Advances in the basic sciences of bone and vascular biology have led to an improved understanding of vascular pathology and calcification, and we have gained an important understanding and appreciation of the extraskeletal manifestations of mineral metabolism.Our diagnostic capabilities have been enhanced through the development of innovative techniques in radiographic imaging and new assay methodologies for PTH and other bone markers. New vitamin D analogs and phosphate binders, as well as calcimimetics, have been added to our therapeutic regimens.

The material in this *Clinical Guide to Bone and Mineral Metabolism in CKD* evolved from the National Kidney Foundation K/DOQI Guidelines for Bone Metabolism and Disease in CKD and was updated to reflect the most current thinking and understanding in this fascinating field. The *Clinical Guide* is specific to the abnormalities in bone and mineral metabolism associated with CKD.

The Clinical Guide was developed to serve the needs of all those who provide care to CKD patients, including nephrologists, nephrology trainees, nephrology nurses and dieticians, cardiologists, endocrinologists, primary care providers, and house officers.

The *Clinical Guide* content covers:

- basic bone and mineral physiology;
- diagnostic approaches, including bone biopsy, imaging techniques and bone biomarkers;
- pathophysiology and clinical manifestations of secondary hyperparathyroidism, renal osteodstrophy, and extraskeletal calcification;
- therapeutic options to manage bone and mineral disorders;
- unique aspects of bone and mineral metabolism in special populations, such as children, patients with hypogonadism, and kidney transplant recipients; and
- epidemiologic data linking abnormalities of bone and mineral metabolism to morbidity and mortality.

Each chapter of the *Clinical Guide* was reviewed by the Editor, co-chairs of GBMI and KDIGO, and two external reviewers. Authors were asked to revise their manuscripts accordingly before acceptance of the manuscripts for inclusion in the text.

I would like to express sincere appreciation to the authors who distilled their knowledge and clinical expertise in this text, and to all those who participated in the review process.

A special note of gratitude goes to Tom Manley for his tireless and skilled editorial work.

I also want to thank the staff of the National Kidney Foundation for their professional management of the project and their technical support in the development of the *Clinical Guide*.

Klaus Olgaard, MD

1

MINERAL HOMEOSTASIS AND BONE PHYSIOLOGY

William G. Goodman
L. Darryl Quarles

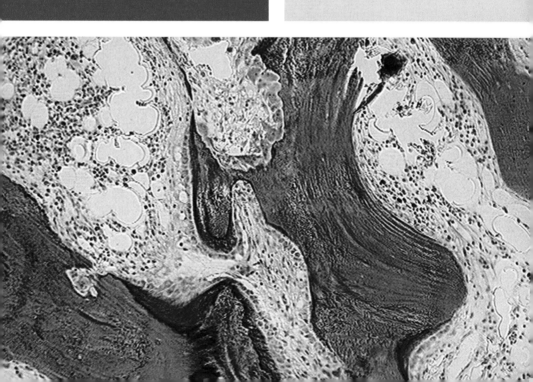

CHAPTER 1

MINERAL HOMEOSTASIS AND BONE PHYSIOLOGY

William G. Goodman and L. Darryl Quarles

Mineral homeostasis, bone metabolism, and kidney function are highly interrelated. The kidneys regulate the net excretion of calcium and phosphorus in the urine and maintain total body balance of both minerals. This is achieved by responding to changes in calcium and phosphorus absorption by the intestines and by modifying ion exchange between extracellular fluid and bone. Bone provides an abundant, endogenous source of calcium and phosphorus to support the metabolic and homeostatic requirements of the body. Parathyroid hormone (PTH), calcitriol, and phosphatonins are the key hormonal factors that coordinate the responses of the kidney, intestine, and bone. The importance of adequate kidney function for maintaining mineral homeostasis and skeletal metabolism is underscored by the prevalence and severity of various disturbances in calcium, phosphorus, and bone that develop during progressive loss of kidney function in patients with chronic kidney disease (CKD).

In order to understand the complex array of bone and mineral disorders that occur with CKD, it is essential to have a thorough understanding of basic bone and mineral biology. This chapter provides an overview of calcium and phosphorus homeostasis, vitamin D metabolism, and normal bone structure, function, and metabolism. The effect of CKD and loss of kidney function on this normal homeostatic process is reviewed in the chapters that follow.

MINERAL HOMEOSTASIS

Calcium

Calcium is the most abundant cation in the body and plays a role in a variety of critical biological processes.[1,2] Calcium salts are a primary structural component of bone and are essential for skeletal integrity. Intracellular and extracellular calcium concentrations affect many biochemical processes that control such activities as skeletal and cardiac muscle contraction, nerve synapse transmission, endocrine function, blood coagulation, and intracellular enzyme activity. As a result, these compartmental calcium concentrations are tightly regulated.

Overview of Calcium Metabolism and the Regulation of Plasma Calcium Levels

More than 99% of calcium resides in bone, whereas less than 1% is found in extracellular fluid (Figure1). Intracellular calcium concentrations are quite low and measurements are expressed in units of micromoles per liter (μmol/L), while the concentration of calcium in extracellular fluid is much higher, with measurements expressed in units of millimoles per liter (mmol/L).

In adults, the skeleton contains approximately 1.2-1.4 kg of elemental calcium, predominantly in the form of hydroxyapatite crystals [$Ca_{10}(PO_4)_6(OH)_2$]. Most calcium in bone serves a structural need. Only a limited amount (approximately 150-200 mg) of skeletal calcium is exchanged daily with the extracellular fluid during the process of skeletal remodeling (Figure 1). However, a separate, more rapidly exchangeable pool of calcium is available to satisfy short-term homeostatic requirements. Calcium influx and efflux from this rapidly exchangeable skeletal pool is influenced by several hormones, including parathyroid hormone (PTH), providing a mechanism to buffer changes in blood calcium concentration.

FIGURE 1. NORMAL CALCIUM HOMEOSTASIS

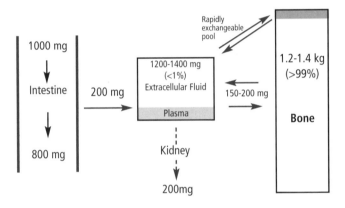

The distribution of calcium in bone and extracellular fluid, and the net amounts of calcium that enter and leave the extracellular fluid each day from bone and the gastrointestinal tract. The movement of calcium between extracellular fluid and a rapidly exchangeable skeletal calcium pool serves to maintain constant levels of ionized calcium in blood and is separate from the amounts exchanged due to ongoing skeletal remodeling. Under steady conditions, calcium excretion in the urine closely approximates net intestinal calcium.

Calcium in extracellular fluids, specifically plasma, exists in three distinct forms. Approximately 40% is bound to plasma proteins, mainly albumin, whereas another 10%-12% forms soluble complexes with various organic anions such as citrate. The most important component of physiological calcium in extracellular fluid is the ionized fraction. It is this portion of calcium in blood that interacts directly with cell membranes, various membrane channels, and the calcium-sensing receptor (CaSR). It is the concentration of ionized calcium in blood that is regulated tightly.

Plasma (or serum) total calcium concentrations in humans range from 8.4-10.2 mg/dL or 2.1-2.6 mmol/L (See Conversion Table in Appendix).* Measurements of plasma total calcium concentration are affected by variations in plasma albumin levels and blood pH. Reductions in

*Values will vary somewhat among reference laboratories due to differences in the methods used for analysis.

plasma albumin concentration diminish the binding of calcium ions to albumin, thus lowering measured values of total plasma calcium concentration. In general, reported values for plasma total calcium decline by approximately 0.8 mg/dL for each 1.0 g/dL decrement in plasma albumin concentration from a reference level of 4.0 g/dL. Reductions in blood pH diminish the albumin-bound fraction of calcium in plasma, resulting in lower measured values for plasma total calcium concentration, while the levels of ionized calcium increase. Conversely, increases in blood pH enhance the albumin-bound fraction of calcium and plasma total calcium levels rise modestly, while the levels of ionized calcium decline. The normal range for blood ionized calcium concentrations in healthy persons is approximately 4.4-5.2 mg/dL (1.1-1.3 mmol/L). Measurements of ionized calcium are useful for assessing calcium metabolism in patients with clinical conditions that affect plasma albumin concentrations, and in those with various acid-base disorders.

Because of the importance of calcium in mediating a wide array of physiological functions, the level of ionized calcium in blood is maintained within a very narrow physiological range. This is accomplished by the coordinated regulation of calcium excretion in the urine to accommodate changes in calcium entry into the extracellular fluid from two primary sources: the gastrointestinal tract and bone (Figure 1). An increase in the reclamation of calcium from tubular fluid, primarily in the distal nephron, provides an additional source of calcium input into the extracellular fluid when intestinal calcium absorption or release from bone is reduced. Conversely, calcium excretion in the urine is enhanced by reductions in calcium reabsorption in both the proximal and distal nephron when excess amounts of calcium enter the extracellular fluid from the gastrointestinal tract or from bone. To a considerable extent, PTH mediates these adaptive changes in renal calcium excretion because the minute-to-minute secretion of PTH is modulated by the CaSR located within the plasma membrane of parathyroid cells.

The CaSR, expressed abundantly in parathyroid tissue, represents the molecular mechanism by which parathyroid cells detect very small changes in ionized calcium concentration and modulate PTH secretion accordingly.[3;4] Reductions in ionized calcium concentration inactivate the CaSR and promote PTH release (Figure 2). Because PTH enhances renal tubular calcium transport in the distal nephron, calcium reabsorption increases and calcium excretion in the urine falls. Increases in PTH secretion also promote calcium mobilization from bone. Both responses occur within minutes to hours and serve to raise blood ionized calcium concentrations toward baseline values. When plasma PTH levels remain elevated for longer periods, 1,25-dihydroxyvitamin D synthesis by the kidney increases and intestinal calcium absorption rises, making more calcium available to correct the calcium level in extracellular fluid.

By contrast, increases in ionized calcium concentration activate the CaSR and inhibit PTH secretion. As a result, renal tubular calcium reabsorption in the distal nephron diminishes, calcium excretion in the urine rises, and less calcium is released from the rapidly exchangeable skeletal calcium pool. Together, these changes serve to lower ionized calcium concentration toward baseline values. With more sustained reductions in plasma PTH levels, renal 1,25-dihydroxyvitamin D production falls and intestinal calcium absorption decreases, reducing the amount of calcium entering extracellular fluid. These adaptive responses to small changes in plasma calcium maintain blood ionized calcium levels within a narrow physiological range. There are likely

FIGURE 2. REGULATION OF PLASMA CALCIUM AND PHOSPHORUS

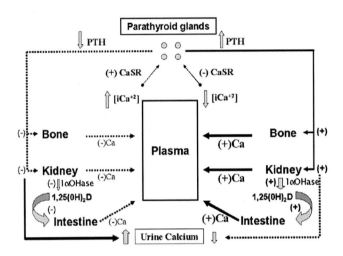

The adaptive responses to a reduction in plasma calcium concentration. Decreases in plasma calcium provoke increased PTH secretion, which, in turn:

1. enhances calcium reabsorption in the distal nephron, thereby reducing calcium excretion in the urine;

2. reduces phosphorus reabsorption in the nephron, thereby increasing phosphorus excretion in the urine;

3. increases bone turnover, thereby mobilizing calcium and phosphorus from bone, and increasing the amount of calcium entering extra-cellular fluid; and

4. stimulates 1α-hydroxylase activity, thereby increasing calcitriol levels and promoting intestinal calcium (and phosphorus) absorption.

All of these actions act to enhance calcium levels in the extracellular fluid, while the increased excretion of phosphorus in the urine acts to maintain normal phosphorus levels. This adaptive process is reversed with increases in plasma calcium levels.

other mechanisms that play a role in minute-to-minute regulation of plasma ionized calcium. Rats that have been parathyroidectomized and nephrectomized are still able to respond rapidly (within minutes) to changes in ionized calcium after acute hypocalcemia is induced.[5]

Calcium Metabolism and Bone

Bone is remodeled continuously throughout much of the skeleton by a tightly regulated sequence of localized cellular events. Groups of osteoclasts initially remove discrete amounts of existing bone during the resorption phase of the skeletal remodeling cycle. Osteoblasts subsequently replace nearly equivalent volumes of bone at each resorption site. In adults, the amounts of calcium and phosphorus mobilized during osteoclastic bone resorption approximate quite closely the amounts replaced by osteoblasts during the formation phase of bone remodeling (Figure 1). Net skeletal calcium and phosphorus balance in adults is thus close to zero. Strictly speaking, however, bone resorption in the adult skeleton slightly exceeds bone formation during each remodeling cycle, and it is this disparity that accounts for age-related bone loss, while the opposite takes place in children with a slightly increased bone formation.

Disorders that enhance the rate of skeletal remodeling, such as hyperparathyroidism and hyperthyroidism, increase the amounts of calcium and phosphorus that are exchanged daily between bone and the extracellular fluid. Conversely, the daily exchange of calcium and phosphorus between bone and extracellular fluid diminishes in clinical conditions that are associated with reduced rates of skeletal remodeling such as hypoparathyroidism. These alterations in bone remodeling may significantly affect long-term bone health, but have little impact on the minute-to-minute regulation of plasma calcium and phosphorus levels. These are affected predominantly by short-term adjustments in mineral flux between plasma and the rapidly exchangeable skeletal mineral pool.

Intestinal Calcium Transport

The transport of calcium by intestinal epithelia occurs by two distinct mechanisms. One is an active, energy-dependent process that regulates the movement of calcium across intestinal epithelial cells. It is affected primarily by vitamin D, and most importantly by its active component, calcitriol (1,25-dihydroxyvitamin D_3). The other is a passive, energy-independent process that traverses the paracellular pathway. This process occurs largely by diffusion, is concentration-dependent, and is unaffected by vitamin D.

The passive, or diffusional, component of intestinal calcium transport is largely unregulated. Approximately 15%-20% of ingested calcium is absorbed by passive mechanisms across a wide range of dietary calcium intakes (RDA of 1,000 mg/d in individuals <50 years and 1,250 mg/d in individuals >50 years). Net calcium absorption via passive mechanisms is small when the dietary intake of calcium is low, but diffusional intestinal calcium absorption, mainly in the duodenum and jejunum, increases progressively as dietary calcium intake rises.

The active transcellular component of calcium absorption in intestinal epithelia is regulated quite tightly, predominantly by calcitriol. Vitamin D-dependent calcium transport represents a crucial response to calcium deprivation, which becomes increasingly important for maintaining net intestinal calcium absorption as dietary calcium intake is reduced. This adaptive response is largely due to an increase in the active, vitamin D-dependent component of intestinal calcium transport that serves to maintain net calcium input into the extracellular fluid at approximately 200 mg/day (Figure 1).

The transcellular movement of calcium in the intestines involves three distinct steps (Figure 3). First, calcium uptake occurs across the apical membrane of intestinal epithelial cells through an epithelial calcium channel (ECaC).[6] Second, calcium entering the cytosol binds to calbindin D_{9K}, a vitamin D-dependent protein.[7] Calbindin D_{9K} appears to act as a transport or shuttle protein that facilitates the movement of calcium ions from the apical brush-border to the basolateral membrane for extrusion from the cell. Also, it probably serves to buffer abrupt increases in cytosolic calcium concentration. Third, calcium extrusion across the basolateral membrane is mediated by a sodium-calcium exchanger (NCX) which is activated by an adenosine triphosphate (ATP)-dependent calcium ATPase (Ca-ATPase).

FIGURE 3. OVERVIEW OF THE TRANSEPITHELIAL MOVEMENT OF CALCIUM IN INTESTINAL AND RENAL TUBULAR EPITHELIAL CELLS

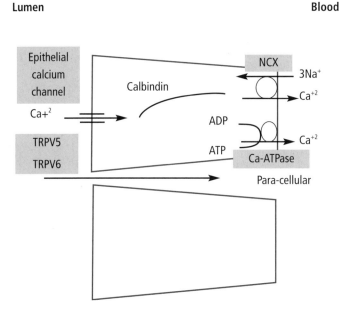

Calcium entry across the apical membrane is mediated by an epithelial calcium channel, predominantly TRPV5 in kidney and TRPV6 in intestine. Calbindin D serves to buffer changes in cytosolic calcium concentration resulting from calcium entry across the apical membrane and facilitates the movement of calcium to the basolateral membrane. Calcium extrusion from the cell is mediated by a sodium-calcium exchanger (NCX) utilizing energy provided by a calcium-ATPase. The levels of expression of calbindin D, TRPV5, and TRPV6 are affected by vitamin D. Calcium transport also occurs passively by diffusion through the paracellular pathway.

Vitamin D has been recognized for many years as a major determinant of intestinal calbindin D_{9K} expression, providing one mechanism to account for vitamin D-mediated increases in intestinal calcium absorption. Recent work indicates, however, that vitamin D also increases calcium entry into cells in calcium-transporting epithelia by upregulating the level of expression of two important members (TRPV5 and TRPV6) of the vanilloid subfamily that are part of the superfamily of transient receptor potential proteins.[8]

Increases in calcitriol production by the kidney are largely responsible for the enhanced efficiency of intestinal calcium transport during dietary calcium restriction. Elevated plasma PTH levels and reductions in plasma calcium concentrations both promote renal 1α-hydroxylase activity, and each probably contributes to this adaptive response. Modest elevations in plasma calcitriol levels enhance the active vitamin D-dependent component of intestinal calcium absorption and optimize the efficiency of intestinal calcium transport, whereas modest elevations in plasma PTH levels also serve to mobilize calcium from bone.

Calcium Transport within the Nephron and Renal Calcium Excretion
In adults in whom net skeletal calcium balance is neutral, the amount of calcium excreted in the urine generally reflects the amount absorbed from the gastrointestinal tract (Figure 1). As described previously, net calcium absorption is approximately 200 mg in vitamin D-replete individuals who ingest diets containing adequate amounts (approximately 1,000 mg/d) of calcium. To maintain total body calcium balance, an equivalent amount of calcium, about 200 mg, must be excreted daily in the urine. The modulation of renal calcium excretion provides an ongoing mechanism to adapt to short-term variations in the amount of calcium entering the extracellular fluid and to maintain constant levels of calcium in plasma. Changes in the efficiency of renal tubular calcium transport, particularly in the distal nephron, mediate this adaptive response.

Parathyroid hormone (PTH) is the major regulator of calcium transport in the distal tubule, promoting tubular calcium reabsorption and diminishing calcium excretion. Other calcium-regulating hormones such as vitamin D and calcitonin have less pronounced effects. The exquisite sensitivity of parathyroid cells to very small changes in ionized calcium concentration allows very rapid changes in PTH secretion to modulate distal tubular calcium transport continuously, and to regulate renal calcium excretion in an ongoing fashion. Other factors that can affect the urinary excretion of calcium via the CaSR, including extracellular calcium itself, are shown in Table 1.

TABLE 1. RENAL CALCIUM EXCRETION

Factors that increase calcium excretion	Factors that decrease calcium excretion
Increased plasma calcium concentration	Decreased plasma calcium concentration
Immobilization	PTH
Low dietary phosphate intake	Thiazide diuretics
Corticosteroid administration	Decreased GFR
Loop diuretics	Increased dietary phosphorus intake
Metabolic acidosis	Amiloride
Increased sodium excretion	

The CaSR is also expressed in the kidney. Inactivating mutations of CaSR result in hypocalci-uria, where activating mutations of the CaSR enhance calcium excretion in the urine. Signaling through the CaSR also affects the renal tubular transport of water and other electrolytes.

Phosphorus

Phosphorus, like calcium, is involved in a wide variety of metabolic and enzymatic processes. Phosphorus is of crucial importance to all biological systems due to its participation in energy metabolism. High-energy phosphate bonds, in the form of ATP, store energy from oxidative reactions. Cyclic AMP is an important high-energy phosphate compound that mediates the intracellular action of many hormones on target cells. Calcium and phosphorus together, as a component of hydroxyapatite, represent the major mineral components of bone and are essential for normal bone mineralization.

Overview of Phosphorus Metabolism

The total body content of phosphorus in adults is approximately 700 g. Phosphorus, like calci-um, is found predominantly in mineralized skeletal tissues in the form of apatite crystals. Phosphorus-containing compounds are, however, important intracellular constituents, and approximately 15% of phosphorus is located in soft tissues, particularly in muscle. Less than 1% of phosphorus is found in extracellular fluid (Figure 4).

FIGURE 4. NORMAL PHOSPHORUS HOMEOSTASIS

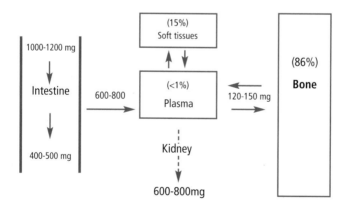

The distribution of phosphorus among bone, soft tissues, and extracellular fluid, and the net amounts of phosphorus entering and leaving the extracellular fluid each day from bone and the gastrointestinal tract. Under steady-state conditions in adults, the amount of phosphorus excreted in the urine each day largely reflects net intestinal phosphorus absorption.

The dietary intake of phosphorus in adults typically ranges from 1,000-1,400 mg/d and is determined largely by the ingested amounts of protein and dairy products. Total body phosphorus balance is generally neutral in healthy adults with normal kidney function. As discussed previously with respect to calcium metabolism, phosphorus excretion in the urine varies primarily as a function of the amounts entering the extracellular fluid from the gastrointestinal tract (Figure 4). The net exchange of phosphorus between bone and soft tissues on the one hand and the extracellular fluid on the other is close to zero under basal conditions.

Normal fasting plasma phosphorus concentration is maintained between 2.5-4.5 mg/dL or 0.81-1.45 mmol/L. Approximately two-thirds of plasma phosphorus is organic. Of primary consideration here is inorganic phosphorus, occurring mainly as HPO_4^{2-} and $H_2PO_4^-$. Inorganic plasma phosphorus can exist as phosphate in its ionized form, bound to protein, or complexed with calcium, sodium, or magnesium. Protein binding is minimal, representing about 10% of the total, while 35%-40% is complexed and the rest is ionized. Thus, about 90% of inorganic plasma phosphorus is ultrafilterable.

Phosphorus Metabolism and Bone

Approximately 125-150 mg of phosphorus enters and leaves the extracellular fluid each day as a result of ongoing skeletal remodeling. In adults, net skeletal phosphorus balance is close to zero in the absence of overt metabolic bone disease. Because the capacity of the kidneys to modify phosphorus excretion in the urine is quite large, variations in the rate of skeletal remodeling and in the amount of phosphorus exchanged daily between bone and the extracellular fluid do not substantially affect plasma phosphorus levels unless kidney function is impaired markedly (GFR <40 mL/min/1.73 m^2). High rates of phosphorus efflux from bone due to secondary hyperparathyroidism may, however, aggravate hyperphosphatemia in patients with little or no residual kidney function who require treatment with dialysis.

Recent studies have identified several factors that play a pivotal role in regulating phosphorus uptake into bone by osteoblasts and in mediating skeletal mineralization.[9] These circulating factors, collectively termed "phosphatonins," appear to be components of a distinct new hormonal/autocrine/paracrine network that not only affects phosphorus metabolism in bone but also regulates phosphorus homeostasis systemically. Recent studies implicate fibroblast growth factor FGF-23, which is produced in bone, as the principle phosphatonin and point to a bone-kidney axis that regulates phosphorus homeostasis. There may also be other "phosphatonins," but the relative importance of each of these factors as modifiers of phosphorus metabolism has yet to be determined.

Intestinal Phosphorus Transport

Between 60% and 70% of dietary phosphorus is absorbed by the gastrointestinal tract. The net input of phosphorus into the extracellular fluid from the gastrointestinal tract is approximately 600-800 mg/day. It is this amount of phosphorus that will be excreted in the urine each day to maintain neutral total body balance (Figure 4).

Intestinal phosphorus absorption is primarily a passive or diffusional process that is concentration-dependent.[10] There is, however, a small energy-dependent component of intestinal phosphorus transport, whereby the uptake of sodium and phosphorus across the apical brush-border membrane of intestinal epithelial cells is mediated by the sodium-phosphate cotransporter (NPT2b), utilizing energy provided by sodium-potassium ATPase (Na/K-ATPase).

The presence of certain constituents within the intestinal lumen retards phosphorus absorption. A high dietary intake of calcium diminishes net intestinal phosphorus absorption by promoting the formation of insoluble complexes of calcium and phosphorus within the intestinal lumen. Other bases, such as aluminum hydroxide, aluminum carbonate, and lanthanum carbonate also bind phosphorus in the lumen of the small intestine and diminish phosphorus absorption. These compounds and calcium-free, phosphate-binding resins (such as sevelamer) are used therapeutically to manage phosphorus retention and to control hyperphosphatemia in patients with CKD.

Vitamin D sterols promote intestinal phosphorus absorption by increasing sodium-phosphate cotransport across the apical brush-border membrane. The effect of vitamin D to enhance intestinal phosphorus absorption is one factor that accounts for the worsening of hyperphosphatemia in many patients with CKD who are given vitamin D sterols to treat secondary hyperparathyroidism.

Phosphorus Transport within the Nephron and Renal Phosphorus Excretion
Most inorganic phosphorus in plasma is in an ultrafilterable form. It thus readily crosses the filtration barrier within the glomerulus and is found in proximal tubular fluid at concentrations similar to those in plasma. Approximately 60%-70% of the filtered load of phosphorus is reabsorbed in the proximal nephron, which serves as the primary site for regulating phosphorus excretion in the urine. Lesser amounts of phosphorus are reabsorbed in more distal nephron segments.

PTH is a potent modifier of renal phosphorus excretion, and can markedly increase renal phosphorus excretion. It acts primarily in the proximal nephron to diminish phosphorus reabsorption, but there is some evidence to suggest that PTH also affects phosphorus transport in the distal nephron. Phosphorus is also regulated by PTH-independent pathways. Fibroblast growth factor 23 (FGF23) is a novel phosphaturic factor identified from genetic studies of autosomal dominant hypophosphatemic rickets (ADHR). FGF23 is also likely involved in the pathogenesis of other hypophosphatemic disorders, such as tumor-induced osteomalacia (TIO), ADHR, X-linked hypophosphatemic rickets (XLH) and McCune-Albright disease. FGF23 is predominiently produced by osteoblasts in bone, but it is expressed at low levels in other tissues. FGF23 targets putative FGF receptors located in the proximal tubule, leading to the inhibition of phosphorus reabsorption and to impaired $1,25(OH)_2D_3$ production. How FGF23-mediated control of renal phosphorus handling and $1,25(OH)_2D_3$ production is integrated with the PTH-vitamin D axis has not been defined.

The effects of calcitriol on phosphorus handling by the kidney have not been defined clearly. Although the administration of calcitriol generally reduces phosphorus excretion in the urine, vitamin D-mediated changes in plasma calcium and plasma PTH levels may be largely responsible for this effect.

Other hormones that affect renal phosphorus excretion include calcitonin, insulin, and glucagon (Table 2). The impact of calcitonin on renal phosphorus excretion is relatively minor. Insulin administration generally reduces phosphorus excretion in the urine, but the anabolic effect of insulin to promote phosphorus uptake into cells may account, at least in part, for this change. Glucagon increases renal phosphorus excretion, whereas hyperglycemia increases phosphorus excretion in the urine as a result of ongoing osmotic diuresis. Diuretic agents that act in the proximal nephron (e.g., acetazolamide) and loop diuretics (e.g., furosemide) may also enhance phosphorus excretion.

TABLE 2. RENAL PHOSPHORUS EXCRETION.

Factors that increase phosphorus excretion	Factors that decrease phosphorus excretion
Increased plasma phosphorus concentration	Decreased plasma phosphorus concentration
PTH	Chronic renal failure
Calcitonin	Growth hormone
Renal tubular disease	Thyroid hormone
Volume expansion	
Metabolic acidosis	
Glucocorticoids	

Vitamin D

Overview of Vitamin D Metabolism

Vitamin D is found in nature in two forms: ergocalciferol (vitamin D_2), which originates from plant sources, and cholecalciferol (vitamin D_3), which originates from animal sources. The biological actions of ergocalciferol and cholecalciferol are essentially the same and their metabolism is quite similar. Dietary sources of vitamin D_3 include fatty fishes, fish oils (such as cod liver oil), and fortified foods (such as milk, cereals, and breads). Apart from dietary sources, vitamin D_3 is also produced in skin, representing an additional endogenous source of this important secosteroid. In man, previtamin D_3 is generated from 7-dehydrocholesterol in the skin during exposure to ultraviolet light. Previtamin D_3 is then converted to vitamin D_3 or cholecalciferol, which is released into the blood where it circulates bound to vitamin D-binding protein (DBP).

Two important hydroxylation steps occur normally in the metabolism of vitamin D, both of which increase its biological activity (Figure 5). The carbon located at the 25-position on the side-chain of native vitamin D undergoes hydroxylation in the liver to form 25-hydroxyvitamin D. This enzymatic step is not regulated tightly, is substrate-dependent, and is unaffected by CKD. Measurements of the plasma level of 25-hydroxyvitamin D thus represent the best index of vitamin D intake, both in the general population and in those with kidney failure. Most 25-hydroxyvitamin D circulates in plasma bound to DBP and only a very small fraction exists in the unbound state.

FIGURE 5. VITAMIN D METABOLISM

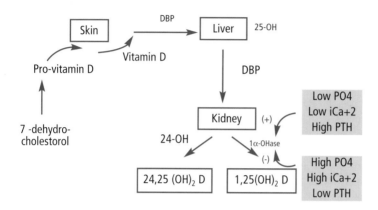

Both vitamin D3 (cholecalciferol) and vitamin D2 (ergocalciferol) circulate in plasma bound to vitamin D-binding protein (DBP) and undergo hydroxylation at the 25-position in the liver. The 25-hydroxylated metabolites then undergo 1α-hydroxylation in the kidney. Calcium, phosphorus and PTH each modify the activity of the renal 1α-hydroxylase independently. The 24-hydroxylation of 25-hydroxyvitamin D probably represents the initial step in the degradation or inactivation of vitamin D.

Calcitriol, or 1,25-dihydroxycholecalciferol, is the biologically most potent metabolite of vitamin D_3 and is formed by the hydroxylation of the carbon located at the first position of the A-ring of 25-hydroxyvitamin D. This step is mediated by a 25-hydroxyvitamin D 1α-hydroxylase, located in cells of the proximal tubule.

The renal production of calcitriol is regulated separately by calcium, phosphorus, FGF-23, and PTH. Low ambient levels of calcium or phosphorus and increases in PTH levels promote renal 1α-hydroxylase activity and enhance calcitriol synthesis (Figure 5). Conversely, high ambient calcium or phosphorus levels, decreases in PTH, and increments in FGF-23 diminish renal 1α-hydroxylase activity.

High plasma calcium levels and conditions of calcium surfeit also promote the activity of another enzyme, the renal 25-hydroxyvitamin D 24-hydroxylase, leading to the formation of 24,25-dihydroxycholecalciferol (Figure 5). This metabolic conversion is generally considered to represent an initial step in the degradation or inactivation of vitamin D and, together with calcium-mediated reductions in renal 1α-hydroxylase activity, diminishes calcitriol production in states of hypercalcemia.

Because renal 1α-hydroxylase activity is regulated tightly, the plasma levels of calcitriol and 25-hydroxyvitamin D are generally unrelated in healthy persons with adequate vitamin D nutrition, and measured values for the two metabolites do not correlate. The availability of 25-

hydroxyvitamin D has little effect on net calcitriol production unless severe vitamin D deficiency has already developed. Renal calcitriol synthesis is maintained in less advanced states of vitamin D deficiency due to increases in renal 1α-hydroxylase activity mediated by hypocalcemia, hypophosphatemia, and elevated plasma PTH levels, either alone or together. Thus, calcitriol levels remain normal—or may even be elevated—despite relatively low plasma levels of 25-hydroxyvitamin D in subjects with mild or moderate vitamin D deficiency. It is for these reasons that plasma 25-hydroxyvitamin D levels, rather than plasma calcitriol concentrations, serve as the best biochemical index of vitamin D status.

In contrast to persons with normal kidney function, the levels of 25-hydroxyvitamin D and calcitriol correlate moderately among patients with CKD. The emergence of this relationship probably reflects disruption of the regulatory control of renal 1α-hydroxylase activity as kidney disease progresses.

Strictly speaking, calcitriol functions as a hormone and fulfills this definition because it is produced locally in a particular tissue, circulates in plasma, and elicits biological responses in remote target tissues. The presence of the 25-hydroxyvitamin D_3 1α-hydroxylase in keratinocytes, cells of the monocyte/macrophage lineage, and bone cells suggests, however, that some tissues regulate calcitriol synthesis locally.

Most of the biological actions of calcitriol are mediated through a genomic mechanism that requires binding of the sterol to the vitamin D receptor (VDR) and subsequent translocation of the ligand-receptor complex to the cell nucleus, where it interacts with the promoter region of various genes. These interactions enhance the expression of some genes such as osteocalcin and the calbindins and diminish the expression of others such as pre-pro-PTH. Because the VDR is expressed quite widely, calcitriol has effects in numerous target tissues.

As discussed previously, vitamin D enhances the movement of calcium and phosphorus across the apical membrane of intestinal epithelial cells.[11] Calcitriol also serves as the major regulator of active intestinal calcium absorption by upregulating the expression of calbindin D_{9K} and other proteins, such as alkaline phosphatase. The mechanisms responsible for increased phosphorus absorption have not been established fully. Most intestinal phosphorus absorption is passive and unregulated; however, it is possible that vitamin D enhances intestinal phosphorus absorption through changes in sodium-phosphate cotransport in intestinal epithelia.

Disturbances in Vitamin D Metabolism due to Kidney Disease

Because the kidneys play such a pivotal role in the production of calcitriol, it is not unexpected that plasma 1,25-dihydroxyvitamin D levels decrease progressively as kidney function declines. Results vary widely, however, among patients at any given level of kidney function, whether judged by measurements of plasma creatinine levels or by estimates of GFR. Technical difficulties with vitamin D assays may account for some of this variation, as well as differences in vitamin D nutrition that may contribute to the range of levels reported. Nevertheless, plasma 1,25-dihydroxyvitamin D levels are normal in some CKD patients, but markedly reduced in others who have only modest reductions in kidney function. Patients whose kidney function has declined to 20%-25% of normal often have quite low plasma calcitriol levels, whereas values may be only modestly reduced in others with a similar degree of impairment in kidney function. The proportion of patients with subnormal plasma calcitriol levels increases, however, as kidney function worsens. Such changes account, at least in part, for reductions in the efficiency of intestinal calcium absorption and for modest decreases in plasma calcium concentration in many patients with CKD Stages 3-4. Indeed, hypocalciuria is a hallmark of moderate renal insufficiency, (CKD Stages 4-5) further emphasizing the importance of adequate renal calcitriol production for maintaining calcium homeostasis in those with progressive kidney disease.

Vitamin D Nutrition and Kidney Disease
Vitamin D nutrition, as indicated by measurements of 25-dihydroxyvitamin D levels in plasma, has been found to be marginal or inadequate both in studies of older persons with osteoporosis[12;13] and in otherwise healthy individuals in the general population.[14-16] Mild secondary hyperparathyroidism and modest elevations in plasma PTH levels are not uncommon, and repletion with vitamin D has been shown to lower plasma PTH levels in older subjects with biochemical evidence of inadequate vitamin D nutrition.[17;18] Such observations serve as the basis for the recent recommendation that patients with CKD should undergo biochemical screening to detect vitamin D deficiency and receive treatment if the disorder is identified.[19]

Although opinions vary somewhat, plasma 25-dihydroxyvitamin D levels between 16-30 ng/mL are considered to reflect marginal vitamin D nutrition, or vitamin D insufficiency.[20] Values ranging from 5-15 ng/mL indicate mild vitamin D deficiency, whereas values <5 ng/mL indicate severe vitamin D deficiency. Vitamin D repletion with ergocalciferol is recommended to restore plasma 25-dihydroxyvitamin D levels to values that exceed 30 ng/mL. The matter of nutritional vitamin D repletion with ergocalciferol is one that should be considered separate and distinct from the use of active vitamin D sterols to treat secondary hyperparathyroidism due to CKD.

It is quite possible that a component of the secondary hyperparathyroidism that emerges as kidney function declines in patients with CKD is due to inadequate vitamin D nutrition, and not solely due to impaired calcitriol production by the diseased kidney. If present, vitamin D insufficiency and/or deficiency are likely to aggravate the disorder. Based upon observations from the general population, inadequate vitamin D nutrition can contribute to the development of secondary hyperparathyroidism in individuals with adequate kidney function, whereas vitamin D repletion can ameliorate the disorder in most or correct it fully in some. Additional work will be required, however, to clarify the role of vitamin D nutrition as a modifier of secondary hyperparathyroidism in patients with CKD Stages 3-4.

Vitamin D and Bone
Vitamin D serves two critical functions in mineralizing tissues. It is an important modulator of cell differentiation and function both for osteoclasts and osteoblasts, and is essential for maintaining the calcification of bone and cartilage.

Calcitriol, or 1,25-dihydroxyvitamin D_3, has major effects on the recruitment and differentiation of osteoclasts. These actions are due largely to calcitriol-induced upregulation of the receptor activator of NF-κB ligand (RANKL) and its cognate receptor RANK that together mediate cell-to-cell interactions between marrow stromal cells and cells of the monocyte-macrophage lineage, which differentiate ultimately into fully mature osteoclasts. Although other cytokines and growth factors also influence osteoclast differentiation, calcitriol plays a critical role in the early recruitment of uncommitted precursors toward osteoclastic differentiation. Calcitriol has much less striking effects on the differentiated functions of mature osteoclasts.

Calcitriol is an important determinant of the levels of expression of selected biochemical markers of osteoblastic differentiation, such as type I collagen, alkaline phosphatase, osteopontin, and osteocalcin at various stages of osteoblastic maturation. Calcitriol may, however, diminish the overall recruitment and/or differentiation of precursors into fully mature osteoblasts and impede differentiated functions in fully mature osteoblasts, including collagen synthesis.

Most experimental evidence indicates that calcitriol supports skeletal mineralization primarily by maintaining adequate concentrations of calcium and phosphorus in extracellular fluid. Most compelling in this regard are data indicating that the calcification of bone and epiphyseal growth plate cartilage is normal in VDR knockout mice if plasma calcium and phosphorus levels are maintained within the normal range by dietary modification.[21] Thus, calcium and phosphorus alone are sufficient to support adequate skeletal mineralization in tissues lacking a functional VDR.

BONE PHYSIOLOGY

Bone Function
The skeletal system provides structural support and protection of internal organs. It is the attachment site for muscles that allows movement. Bone is the primary reservoir for the critical minerals, calcium and phosphorus, and for carbonate and phosphate salts that provide a long-term supply of buffer, especially during prolonged metabolic acidosis.

Bone Structure
The organic matrix of bone is composed primarily of protein collagen fibers that provide flexibility. Interspersed in the matrix and in varying density are crystals of hydroxyapatite, an insoluble complex of calcium and phosphate. Bone also contains small amounts of magnesium, sodium, and bicarbonate.

Macro-architecture
There are two major bone types in the human skeleton: cortical (compact) and trabecular (spongy or cancellous; see Figure 6) Cortical bone is a dense layer of calcified tissue that forms the protective outer shell around all bone and is the exclusive component in the midshaft of long bones. It provides structural strength. Nearly 80% of the total skeletal mass is from cortical bone. Cortical bone is organized in a series of parallel and overlapping "bull's eyes" referred to as osteons or Haversian systems. Each osteon contains a central vascular channel surrounded by a concentric space (the Haversian canal), which is in turn surrounded by layers of mineralized bone, the lamellae. The Haversian canal contains capillaries, arterioles, venules, and nerves.

FIGURE 6. SCHEMATIC VIEW OF A LONGITUDINAL SECTION THROUGH A GROWING BONE

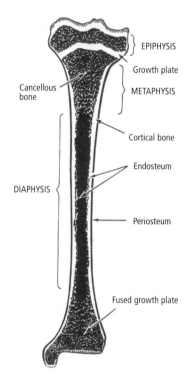

Reproduced with permission from Baron, R. (1999). Anatomy and ultrastructure of bone. In M.J.Favus (Ed.), Primer on metabolic bone diseases and disorders of mineral metabolism (4 ed., pp. 3-10). Philadelphia: Lippincott Williams and Wilkens.

Trabecular bone provides the interior supporting structure of bone. It can be described as an intricate web made of bone plates or rods with many interposed sinuses that are filled with bone marrow, mesenchymal cells, and other tissues. It provides a rigid internal scaffolding to maintain the bone's shape despite significant compressive forces. It constitutes only 20% of total bone mass, but—due to its multiple sinuses—constitutes 80% of the total bone surface area. It is found in the epiphyseal and metaphyseal regions of long bone and throughout the interior of short bone, constituting the majority of the axial skeleton, the ribs, spine, and skull.

The outer surface of bone is covered by a tough, fibrous membrane, the periosteum. The endosteum is comprised of layers of cells that line the inner cavity of bones.

Micro-architecture

Bone is formed and maintained by living bone cells that are interspersed throughout the tissue. Bone cells are divided into two major categories: osteoclasts and osteoblasts. In general, osteoclasts are the cells that resorb bone and osteoblasts are cells that deposit bone.

FIGURE 7. OSTEOGENESIS

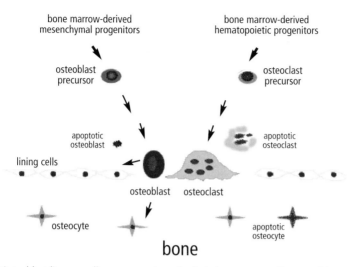

Osteoblast lineage cells are mesenchymal cells in bone marrow. The osteoblast precursor cells go through several phases to differentiate into mature osteoblasts. This differentiation is affected by various factors, such as Cbfa 1. The mature osteoblasts lay down proteins on the bone surface that will form the organic matrix of bone and lead to mineralization. Once the osteoblasts complete bone production some will differentiate into osteocytes and be incorporated into the bone matrix. Others will differentiate into bone lining cells. Osteoclasts share lineage with blood cells, particularly macrophages. Mature osteoclasts are formed from the fusion of precursor cells under the control of RANKL and osteoprotegerin. Osteoclasts secrete acids and enzymes to resorb bone. Osteoclasts activity ends when they undergoing apoptosis. Reproduced with permission from: Ott, S. M., Bruder, J. M. (Eds) (2004). Bone Curriculum. ASBMR. [On-Line]. Available: **http://depts.washington.edu/bonebio/ASBMRed/ASBMRed.html**

Osteoclasts

Osteoclasts secrete enzymes and acids that break down *or resorb* mineralized bone. They are large, irregularly shaped cells that are frequently multinucleated. The cell membrane has multiple folds and invaginations in the area that abuts the bone surface. This enhances contact with the bone and is referred to as the ruffled border.

It is along ruffled border of osteoclasts that resorption occurs. The proteolytic enzymes released by osteoclasts digest collagen and release minerals into the bloodstream. They create minute erosions on the bone surface, called Howship's lacunae.

These unique, highly specialized cells are localized on endosteal surfaces, in Haversian systems and, less frequently, on periosteal surfaces. They are commonly located where there is active bone remodeling such as at the ends of bones beneath epiphyseal growth plate cartilages.

Osteoclasts arise from hematopoietic mononuclear cells in the bone marrow (Figure 7). Their precursors circulate in the blood and arise from bone marrow. Once their bone resorptive activity is complete, they separate from the bone surface and undergo apoptosis, a programmed cell death that is partially regulated by proteins from other cells.

Osteoblasts

Osteoblasts are the bone-building or bone-forming cells. They are cuboidal or columnar in shape and are mononuclear. Their cellular structure is typical of metabolically active cells, with an extensive network of endoplasmic reticulum in the cytosol closest to the adjacent bone surface. Another characteristic of osteoblasts is the presence of large amounts of the enzyme alkaline phosphatase that is secreted during osteoblastic activity.

Osteoblasts form and secrete collagen fibrils which intertwine to form fibers of the bone matrix, the osteoid. The next step in bone formation is the precipitation of calcium and phosphorus salts from the blood. This process is not fully understood, but is at least partially under the influence of osteoblasts. These minerals then bond to form hydroxyapatite crystals that infiltrate the newly formed osteoid to create mineralized bone.

Osteoblasts originate from bone marrow precursor cells (Figure 6). They are then induced to become osteoprogenitor cells, then endosteal or periosteal progenitor cells, and then mature osteoblasts. This differentiation pathway is controlled in early stages by bone morphogenic proteins and the transcription factor Cbfa1, and later by other hormones and cytokines.

Osteoblasts that become embedded in osteoid are called osteocytes. They no longer actively form bone, but remain connected through a network of canaliculi and are thought to play a role in a cellular feedback mechanism, and in the minute-to-minute control of plasma calcium and phosphorus. Osteoblasts also become bone-lining cells, which are flat, pancake-shaped cells that line the entire surface of bone. Bone-lining cells are responsible for the immediate release of calcium and phosphorus, and protect bone from plasma chemicals that can dissolve bone.

SKELETAL GROWTH

Bone Modeling

During childhood, long bones grow both in length and diameter. Longitudinal growth is dependent on the proliferation of cartilage cells in the epiphyseal growth plate at both the proximal and distal ends of long bones. During growth, there is a continual process along each growth plate in which chondrocytes proliferate, mature, hypertrophy, and eventually die (Figure 8). The area around the apoptotic chondrocytes then undergoes a process of matrix formation and mineralization. This process is influenced by multiple hormones and local factors. Ultimately, the balance between proliferation and maturation shifts towards maturation after puberty, and the area of proliferating chondrocytes declines until the epiphysis fuses and the growth plate is eliminated. Long bones also grow in diameter through a process of appositional growth beneath the periosteal surface. Bone remodeling takes place simultaneously with these growth processes.[22]

Acquisition of Bone Mass

The accumulation of calcium in the skeletal system begins at birth and continues unabated until the epiphyseal growth plate cartilages close at the end of adolescence, when the acquisition of peak adult bone mass is nearly complete. This osteoid mineralization is dependent on adequate levels of extracellular calcium and phosphorus, and net calcium retention is quite

FIGURE 8. BONE REMODELING

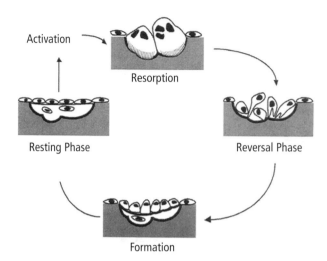

The bone-remodeling sequence as it occurs in trabecular bone. (The same principles apply to Haversian remodeling.) Reproduced with permission from the American Society for Bone and Mineral Research Baron R 2003 General Principles of Bone Biology In: Favus M (ed.) The Primer on the Metabolic Bone Diseases and Disorders of Mineral Metabolism, 5th ed. American Society for Bone and Mineral Research. Washington DC, USA, pp. 1-8. Schematic representation of the cellular events occurring at the growth plate in long bones. R, resorption; Rev, reversal; F, formation; CC, calcified cartilage; WB, woven bone; LB, lamellar bone.

high during periods of rapid bone growth. The accumulation of calcium is most profound during puberty and corresponds to an increase in the levels of calcitriol and other enzymes associated with increased bone turnover and mineralization.[23]

The primary modeling of bones during skeletal growth occurs at sites distinct from those at which existing bone is being remodeled, and the factors that modulate these two processes differ fundamentally.

Bone Remodeling
Bone is continually being renewed by remodeling.[24] Bone remodeling or turnover occurs predominantly on bone surfaces, and the turnover rate is proportional to the number of active remodeling units in any given area. Trabecular bone, with its large surface to mass ratio (20% of the total mass but 80% of the total surface area), is the predominant site of bone remodeling. Bone turnover is affected by a large number of variables, including sex, age, and a variety of hormonal and local factors.

Bone remodeling involves two contrasting activities: resorption and formation. This process occurs at multiple sites throughout the skeletal system, in bone remodeling units made up of osteoclasts and osteoblasts. The remodeling sequence starts with activation, frequently in response to bone micro-damage or mechanical stress. Osteoclasts begin the active process by dissolving bone matrix and collagen, thus clearing away old or damaged bone. Osteoblasts subsequently move in to synthesize bone matrix and simulate mineralization, thus filling the cavity with newly formed bone. (Figure 9)

To maintain healthy bone, it is critical that resorption and formation occur in a coordinated fashion. Regulation of bone remodeling is a complex process involving multiple systemic hormones and local factors. Osteoblasts, which express PTH, vitamin D, and other receptors, serve a pivotal functional role in controlling bone formation and resorption, and in integrating systemic calcium and phosphorus homeostasis with the maintenance of bone mass. Local factors are molecules produced by skeletal cells that communicate with other nearby cells. These factors affect cells of osteoclast and osteoblast lineage by controlling their proliferation, differentiation, recruitment, and survival. Systemic hormones can have direct or indirect effects on bone cells by controlling the synthesis, activation, receptor binding, and protein binding of the local growth factors.

FIGURE 9. BONE GROWTH AND REMODELING AT THE EPIPHYSEAL PLATE

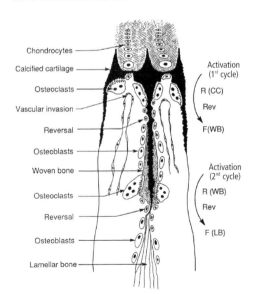

Schematic representation of the cellular events occuring at the growth plate in long bones. R, resorption; Rev, reversal; F, formation; CC, calcified cartilage; WB, woven bone; LB, lamellar bone. Reproduced with permission from: Baron, R. (1999). Anatomy and ultrastructure of bone. In M.J.Favus (Ed.), Primer on metabolic bone diseases and disorders of mineral metabolism (4 ed., pp. 3-10). Philadelphia: Lippincott Williams and Wilkens.

Local Regulators

A number of local factors have been identified that act on bone-related cells to either stimulate or inhibit osteoclastic and osteoblastic activity. They are critical to the initiation of bone remodeling and the normal coupling of resorption and formation.

Growth Factors
- Bone morphogenetic proteins (BMPs) are produced in the bone and bone marrow. They affect the production of Cbfa 1 (also called Runx2), a gene transcription factor that stimulates mesenchymal stem cells in the bone marrow to differentiate into mature osteoblasts.[25;26] BMPs increase bone formation and may decrease resorption; they are currently under investigation as possible therapeutic agents in the treatment of renal osteodystrophy.[27]

- Insulin-like growth factors (IGFs) are synthesized in multiple tissues, including bone.[26;28] Osteoblasts produce IGFs in response to hormones, such as PTH and estrogen, or BMPs. IGFs enhance bone collagen and matrix formation and stimulate osteoblast cellular division, thus increasing the number of new cells. They may also induce osteoblastic differentiation.

- Transforming growth factor-β (TGF-β) is a polypeptide that is released from the bone matrix during osteoclastic bone resorption and has osteoblast-stimulating properties.[24]

Cytokines
- Interleukin-1 (IL-1), interleukin-6 (IL-6), and tumor necrosis factor (TNF) are produced by osteoblastic cells in response to systemic regulators (discussed in the following section). They effect differentiation of bone marrow stem cells into preosteoclasts, inhibit apoptosis in osteoblasts, and cause changes in the proliferation and differentiation of osteoblasts.[26]

- Osteoprotegerin (OPG) and the receptor-activator of the nuclear factor κB system (RANK) play an essential role in osteoclast function and the coupling of osteoclast and osteoblast activities.[29] RANK is a membrane receptor located on preosteoclast cells. When activated by RANK ligand (RANKL), the RANK receptors promote the differentiation of preosteoclast cells into mature osteoclasts, thus stimulating bone resorption. RANKL is secreted by the bone-lining cells under the influence of other local systemic regulators, such as IL-1, calcitriol, and PTH. RANKL is also secreted by osteoblast precursors. OPG is a decoy receptor that can bind the RANK ligand and prevent it from activating the RANK receptor, thereby reducing osteoclastogenesis and bone resorption. The balance or ratio of OPG to RANKL is therefore critical to the relative balance in bone formation and resorption. Understanding this system has led to important research on pharmacological measures to reduce bone loss by altering the OPG to RANKL ratio. The OPG/RANK/RANKL system has also been implicated in the development of vascular disease, discussed in more detail in Chapter 4. This control system is regulated by nearly every cytokine and hormone considered important in bone remodeling, including PTH, 1,25-dihydroxyvitamin D, estrogen, glucocorticoids, interleukins, prostaglandins, and members of the TGF-β superfamily of cytokines.

Systemic Regulators

Many of the classical hormones from the thyroid, adrenal, pituitary, and parathyroid glands affect bone metabolism.[26]

- The primary function of PTH is to maintain calcium homeostasis by means of its actions on the rate of renal reabsorption of calcium and the synthesis of calcitriol. The direct effect of PTH on bone is to stimulate osteoclastic bone resorption. Bone formation that is coupled with this resorption is also increased.[26] During embryonic development, parathyroid hormone-related peptide (PTHrP) plays a role in chondrocyte differentiation. Its function in adult bone physiology is not clear, but it may act locally to promote bone cell differentiation.[30]

- Calcitonin is a peptide hormone secreted by the C-cells in the thyroid gland in response to high plasma calcium concentrations.[31] Calcitonin functions to lower plasma calcium by: 1) inhibiting osteoclastic resorption; 2) reducing calcium absorption in the intestine; and 3) reducing renal calcium reabsorption.

- Vitamin D in its active form, calcitriol, is a hormone that—in addition to its effects on calcium and phosphorus, as previously described—may have a direct effect on bone by enhancing osteoclast formation.

- Insulin stimulates bone matrix synthesis and cartilage formation, and has a marked effect on normal skeletal growth. It is also necessary for normal bone mineralization.

- Gonadal steroids (estrogens and androgens) play an important role in skeletal maturation in growing individuals, and in maintaining bone health. Receptors have been identified for both estrogen and testosterone on bone, but their exact mechanism of action is unclear. Both classes of steroids help regulate the rates of bone formation and resorption and are important for normal bone strength. Reductions in gonadal steroids with aging and menopause contribute to progressive reduction in bone density common in the elderly.

- Glucocorticoids have marked effects on bone and mineral metabolism. Their actions on bone and mineral include: 1) decreased intestinal calcium absorption; 2) reduced bone formation; 3) increased bone resorption; and 4) increased renal calcium excretion. Excess glucocorticoid levels can have significant deleterious effect on bone.

- Thyroid hormone is necessary for normal growth and maturation of the skeleton, primarily through its actions on cartilage formation. The predominant action on bone is to increase osteoclastic bone resorption. Elevated thyroid hormone levels can result in hypercalcemia and enhance osteoporosis.

- Growth hormone (GH) appears to be important in maintaining normal bone mass. Its mechanism of action is not clear but it may indirectly stimulate bone formation, partially by stimulating the production of IGFs. It is critical for longitudinal bone growth during childhood and adolescence.

- The sympathetic nervous system may also regulate bone mass through the β-adrenergic receptor 2 (Arb2) located in osteoblasts. Stimulation of Arb2 results in bone loss, whereas inhibition of this receptor is associated with increased bone mass.

- FGF23 is also involved in regulation of skeletal development. FGF23 null mice have abnormal skeletogenesis, whereas excess FGF23 is associated with rickets and osteomalacia. Patients with CKD have increased circulating FGF23 levels, but the role of this factor in the pathogenesis of renal osteodystrophy remains to be defined.

Mechanism of Bone Loss

Both quality (strength) and quantity (density) need to be considered when evaluating bone. Bone quality/strength is primarily a function of trabecular microstructure, whereas bone quantity/density is a measure of the degree of mineralization. During childhood and teenage years, bone formation exceeds bone resorption. As a result, bones become larger, heavier, and denser. Bone formation continues at a pace faster than resorption until peak bone mass is reached around age 30. After that, bone resorption slowly begins to exceed bone formation during each remodeling cycle, and it is this disparity that accounts for age-related bone loss. The degree of bone loss is influenced by a number of factors, including nutrition, genetics, age, race, gender, body size, activity levels, and medication use.

CONCLUSIONS

As detailed in this chapter, normal bone and mineral metabolism is dependent on a complex regulatory interplay of paracrine, endocrine, and renal functions. The overview presented here provides a glimpse into the basic processes involved in maintaining a delicate balance among levels of calcium, phosphorus, PTH, and vitamin D. The section on bone physiology highlights the physiological factors involved in bone formation and resorption. The disruption of these regulatory pathways by progressive kidney disease accounts for the increased prevalence and severity of bone and mineral disturbances in patients with CKD, and is the subject of the following chapters.

REFERENCES

1. Broadus AE: Mineral balance and homeostasis, in Favus MJ (ed): Primer on metabolic bone diseases and disorders of mineral metabolism, chap 12. Philadelphia, 1999, pp 74-80

2. Heaney RP: Calcium, in Bilezikian JP, Raisz LG, Rodan GA (eds): Principles of Bone Biology, chap 72. San Diego, 1996, pp 1007-1018

*3. Brown EM, Pollak M, Hebert SC: The extracellular calcium-sensing receptor: its role in health and disease. Annu Rev Med 49:15-29, 1998

*4. Chen RA, Goodman WG: Role of the calcium-sensing receptor in parathyroid gland physiology. Am J Physiol Renal Physiol 286:F1005-F1011, 2004

5. Lewin E, Wang W, Olgaard K: Rapid recovery of plasma ionized calcium after acute induction of hypocalcaemia in parathyroidectomized and nephrectomized rats. Nephrol Dial Transplant 14:604-609, 1999

6. Hoenderop JG, Nilius B, Bindels RJ: ECaC: the gatekeeper of transepithelial Ca2+ transport. Biochim Biophys Acta 1600:6-11, 2002

*7. Wasserman RH, Fullmer CS: On the molecular mechanism of intestinal calcium transport. Adv Exp Med Biol 249:45-65, 1989

*8. den Dekker E, Hoenderop JG, Nilius B, Bindels RJ: The epithelial calcium channels, TRPV5 & TRPV6: from identification towards regulation. Cell Calcium 33:497-507, 2003

9. Quarles LD: FGF23, PHEX, and MEPE regulation of phosphate homeostasis and skeletal mineralization. Am J Physiol Endocrinol Metab 285:E1-E9, 2003

*10. Drezner M: Phosphorus homeostasis and related disorders, in Bilezikian JP, Raisz LG, Rodan GA (eds): Principles of Bone Biology, chap 20. San Diego, 1996, pp 263-276

11. Heaney RP, Barger-Lux MJ, Dowell MS, Chen TC, Holick MF: Calcium absorptive effects of vitamin D and its major metabolites. J Clin Endocrinol Metab 82:4111-4116, 1997

12. Lips P: Vitamin D deficiency and secondary hyperparathyroidism in the elderly: consequences for bone loss and fractures and therapeutic implications. Endocr Rev 22:477-501, 2001

13. Lips P, Duong T, Oleksik A, Black D, Cummings S, Cox D, Nickelsen T: A global study of vitamin D status and parathyroid function in postmenopausal women with osteoporosis: baseline data from the multiple outcomes of raloxifene evaluation clinical trial. J Clin Endocrinol Metab 86:1212-1221, 2001

14. Chapuy MC, Preziosi P, Maamer M, Arnaud S, Galan P, Hercberg S, Meunier PJ: Prevalence of vitamin D insufficiency in an adult normal population. Osteoporos Int 7:439-443, 1997

15. Kauppinen-Makelin R, Tahtela R, Loyttyniemi E, Karkkainen J, Valimaki MJ: A high prevalence of hypovitaminosis D in Finnish medical in- and outpatients. J Intern Med 249:559-563, 2001

16. Romagnoli E, Caravella P, Scarnecchia L, Martinez P, Minisola S: Hypovitaminosis D in an Italian population of healthy subjects and hospitalized patients. Br J Nutr 81:133-137, 1999

17. Khaw KT, Sneyd MJ, Compston J: Bone density parathyroid hormone and 25-hydroxyvitamin D concentrations in middle aged women. BMJ 305:273-277, 1992

18. Ooms ME, Roos JC, Bezemer PD, van der Vijgh WJ, Bouter LM, Lips P: Prevention of bone loss by vitamin D supplementation in elderly women: a randomized double-blind trial. J Clin Endocrinol Metab 80:1052-1058, 1995

19. National Kidney Foundation: K/DOQI clinical practice guidelines for bone metabolism and disease in chronic kidney disease. Am J Kidney Dis 42:1-201, 2003

20. Chapuy MC, Meunier PJ: Vitamin D insufficiency in adults and the elderly, in Feldman D, Glorieux FH, Pike JW (eds): Vitamin D, San Diego, CA, 2004, pp 679-693

21. Li YC, Amling M, Pirro AE, Priemel M, Meuse J, Baron R, Delling G, Demay MB: Normalization of mineral ion homeostasis by dietary means prevents hyperparathyroidism, rickets, and osteomalacia, but not alopecia in vitamin D receptor-ablated mice. Endocrinology 139:4391-4396, 1998

22. Baron R: Anatomy and ultrastructure of bone, in Favus MJ (ed): Primer on the metabolic bone diseases and disorders of mineral metabolism, chap 1. Philadelphia, PA, 1999, pp 3-10

23. Aksnes L, Aarskog D: Plasma concentrations of vitamin D metabolites in puberty: effect of sexual maturation and implications for growth. J Clin Endocrinol Metab 55:94-101, 1982

*24. Mundy GR: Bone remodeling, in Favus MJ (ed): Primer on metabolic bone diseases and disorders of mineral metabolism, chap 4. Philadelphia, 1999, pp 30-38

25. Onishi T, Ishidou Y, Nagamine T, Yone K, Imamura T, Kato M, Sampath TK, ten Dijke P, Sakou T: Distinct and overlapping patterns of localization of bone morphogenetic protein (BMP) family members and a BMP type II receptor during fracture healing in rats. Bone 22:605-612, 1998

26. Ott, S. M. and Bruder, J. M. Eds. Bone Curriculum. American Society of Bone and Mineral Research. 9-29-2004. Ref Type: Electronic Citation

*27. Li T, Surendran K, Zawaideh MA, Mathew S, Hruska KA: Bone morphogenetic protein 7: a novel treatment for chronic renal and bone disease. Curr Opin Nephrol Hypertens 13:417-422, 2004

28. Lian JB, Stein GS, Canalis E, Gehron Robey P, Boskey AL: Bone formation: Oseoblast lineage cells, growth factors, matrix proteins, and the mineralization process, in Favus MJ (ed): Primer on metabolic bone diseases and disorders of mineral metabolism, chap 3. Philadelphia, 1999, pp 14-29

29. Hofbauer LC, Schoppet M: Clinical implications of the osteoprotegerin/RANKL/RANK system for bone and vascular diseases. JAMA 292:490-495, 2004

30. Moseley JM, Martin TJ: Parathyroid hormone-related protein: physiologic actions, in Bilezikian JP, Raisz LG, Rodan GA (eds): Principles of Bone Biology, chap 26. San Diego, 1996, pp 363-376

31. Deftos LJ, Weisman MH, Williams GW, Karpf DB, Frumar AM, Davidson BJ, Parthemore JG, Judd HL: Influence of age and sex on plasma calcitonin in human beings. N Engl J Med 302:1351-1353, 1980

*Suggested Reading

2

PATHOPHYSIOLOGY AND CLINICAL MANIFESTATIONS OF RENAL OSTEODYSTROPHY

Arnold Felsenfeld

Justin Silver

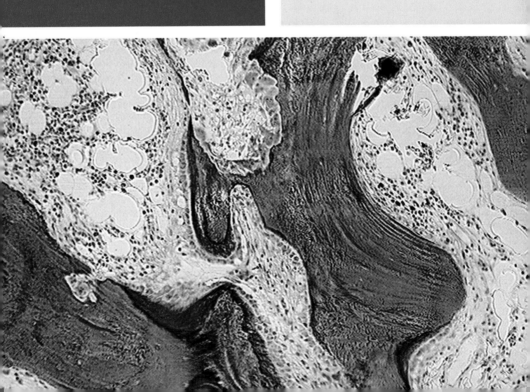

CHAPTER 2

PATHOPHYSIOLOGY AND CLINICAL MANIFESTATIONS OF RENAL OSTEODYSTROPHY

Arnold Felsenfeld and Justin Silver

Secondary hyperparathyroidism (SHPT) and renal osteodystrophy (ROD) are common complications of chronic kidney disease (CKD). These complex, multifactorial disorders have a significant impact on outcomes in patients with kidney disease. It is important for clinicians caring for patients with CKD to understand the factors that contribute to these disorders. This chapter provides a basic review of the pathogenesis and clinical manifestations of SHPT and ROD that occur with CKD.

RENAL OSTEODYSTROPHY

Classification
Renal osteodystrophy is the term used to describe the various skeletal abnormalities that are seen in association with CKD. The classification of ROD is based on histological findings (Table 1). High-turnover bone disease, which is characterized by abnormal and increased bone remodeling, includes osteitis fibrosa and mixed disorders. Low-turnover bone disease, described as decreased bone mineralization and formation, includes osteomalacia and adynamic bone disorder.

HIGH-TURNOVER BONE DISEASE

Secondary Hyperparathyroidism
The vast majority of CKD patients on dialysis have some degree of SHPT that begins in the early stages of CKD and progresses as CKD advances.[2] The development of SHPT results from multiple factors including deficiency of calcitriol, retention of phosphorus, a decrease in expression of the calcium-sensing receptor (CaSR) in the parathyroid gland, and skeletal resistance to the calcemic action of PTH (Table 2).[3-5] In the classic trade-off hypothesis, it was postulated that, as kidney function declines, phosphorus excretion is reduced, plasma phosphorus levels increase, and plasma calcium and calcitriol levels decline. Decreases in calcitriol levels also contribute to a reduction in intestinal calcium absorption. All of these factors contribute to the development of hypocalcemia, which is the primary stimulus for the increased production and secretion of PTH.[5] The subsequent increase in PTH levels stimulates phosphorus excretion and calcitriol production, and corrects the hypocalcemia.[6] At advanced stages of CKD, increased PTH production can no longer prevent the development of hyperphosphatemia and calcitriol deficiency (Figure 1). In animal studies from the 1990s, it was shown that when

TABLE 1. HISTOLOGICAL CLASSIFICATION OF RENAL OSTEODYSTROPHY

Type of Bone Disease	Description	Pathogenesis
High-turnover		
Osteitis fibrosa	Increased bone resorption	SHPT
	Disorganized non-lamellar collagen deposition	
	Increased osteoid deposition	
	Increased rate of bone formation	
	Marrow fibrosis	
Low-turnover		
Osteomalacia	Decreased osteoid deposition	Excess aluminum exposure frequent
	Aluminum accumulation often present	Other unknown factors
	Decreased bone formation rate	
	Accumulation of osteoid because osteoid deposition exceeds bone formation rate	
Adynamic	Few remodeling sites and low bone formation rate	Aluminum deposition sometimes present
	Decreased osteoid deposition	Relatively low PTH levels
		More common in older patients, diabetics, and CAPD patients
High- and low-turnover		
Mixed disease	Increased remodeling sites and resorption activity	SHPT, aluminum deposition, other unknown factors
	Areas of low bone formation	
	Increased osteoid seam width	

Abbreviations: CAPD, continuous ambulatory peritoneal dialysis; SHPT, secondary hyperparathyroidism

TABLE 2. FACTORS CONTRIBUTING TO SECONDARY HYPERPARATHYROIDISM

Hypocalcemia

Hyperphosphatemia (phosphate retention)

Calcitriol deficiency

Impaired skeletal response to PTH

Increased chief cell proliferation (parathyroid glands)

Altered degradation of PTH

Abnormal regulation of calcium-dependent PTH secretion (abnormal set point)

Abbreviation: PTH, parathyroid hormone.

FIGURE 1. PATHOGENESIS OF SECONDARY HYPERPARATHYROIDISM

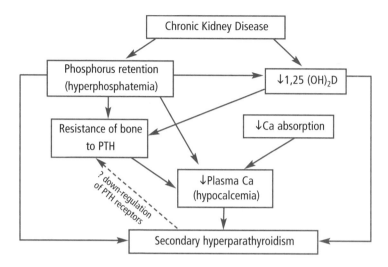

an amount of PTH sufficient to maintain normal plasma calcium, phosphorus, and calcitriol levels in parathyroidectomized rats with normal kidney function was infused into azotemic rats, plasma calcium and calcitriol values decreased and plasma phosphorus values increased.[6] This shows that a greater PTH level is needed in kidney failure to maintain normal mineral homeostasis. In another study, it was shown that as progressive reduction in glomerular filtration rate (GFR) was induced in rats, PTH values progressively increased to maintain normal plasma calcium, phosphorus, and calcitriol levels.[7] Both of these studies lend support to the concepts advanced by the trade-off hypothesis. The abnormalities in phosphorus, calcitriol, and PTH are discussed individually in the following sections.

Phosphorus Retention

Phosphorus retention is one of the key factors in the pathogenesis of SHPT. There are four proposed mechanisms for the effect of phosphorus retention on SHPT. These are: 1) phosphorus-induced hypocalcemia; 2) phosphorus-induced decrease in calcitriol levels; 3) a direct effect of phosphorus on PTH secretion; and 4) a decreased skeletal response to PTH, due to phosphorus retention and hyperphosphatemia.[8]

As GFR decreases in progressive CKD, inadequate phosphorus excretion eventually results in an increase in plasma phosphorus levels. Increases in PTH levels enhance phosphorus excretion by decreasing phosphorus reabsorption in the proximal tubule and restore plasma phosphorus levels to normal. A new steady state is achieved with a higher level of circulating PTH, until the increases in PTH can no longer compensate for the consequences of advanced CKD.[4]

Phosphorus is an important regulator of the production rate of calcitriol. The retention of phosphorus probably decreases the synthesis of calcitriol. Conversely, phosphorus restriction acts to stimulate calcitriol production. While increases in calcitriol during phosphorus restriction may help to prevent hyperparathyroidism or decrease established hyperparathyroidism,[8] studies in animals have shown a calcitriol-independent effect of phosphorus restriction on parathyroid function.

In uremic animals, the effect of plasma phosphorus on PTH gene expression and plasma PTH levels have been shown to be independent of changes in plasma calcium or calcitriol. In studies of dietary phosphorus restriction in which dietary calcium was adjusted to maintain ionized calcium values within the normal range, calcitriol values remained low and did not change. Even though ionized calcium and calcitriol levels did not change, a reduction in the PTH level was noted.[4] Phosphorus also leads to marked changes in parathyroid cell proliferation, increasing with hyperphosphatemia and decreasing with hypophosphatemia.[8]

Decreased Synthesis of Calcitriol

Calcitriol, the active hormonal metabolite of vitamin D, is primarily produced in the proximal tubule of the kidney. Decreased synthesis of calcitriol contributes to the development of SHPT. Plasma calcitriol levels remain in the normal range until the GFR falls to less than 50% of normal. The consequences of low calcitriol levels include direct effects on both the parathyroid gland and the intestine. In the parathyroid glands, calcitriol acts via the vitamin D receptor (VDR) to suppress PTH secretion.[5] In the intestine, low calcitriol levels result in impaired intestinal calcium absorption, thus contributing to hypocalcemia, which—in turn—stimulates PTH secretion.[4]

Altered Parathyroid Function

The parathyroid gland produces, stores, and releases PTH in response to changes in plasma levels of calcium. The response to changes in the plasma calcium concentration is mediated by CaSRs within the parathyroid gland.[5] The VDR also responds to calcitriol. As CKD progresses, hypocalcemia, phosphorus retention, and calcitriol deficiency directly or indirectly stimulate the parathyroid gland to increase production of PTH. This initially leads to parathyroid cell hypertrophy; however, with chronic stimulation, parathyroid cells proliferate and diffuse hyperplasia develops. This proliferation in the number of parathyroid cells is thought to be irreversible and makes control of increased PTH secretion more difficult. With long-term parathyroid stimulation, the proliferating cells often form nodules of abnormal cells within the gland.[9] In areas of nodular hyperplasia, the proliferating cells have been shown to have fewer CaSRs and VDRs.[10;11] Nodular hyperplasia is characterized by resistance to vitamin D therapy, which is at least partly related to the decrease in VDRs and CaSRs.[3] In CKD, there may be a shift in the set-point for calcium-regulated PTH secretion, and the responsiveness to calcium may be altered.[8] While vitamin D receptors are decreased in hyperplastic parathyroid glands, the density of vitamin D receptors is even lower in nodular hyperplasia than in diffuse hyperplasia.[10]

Calcitriol is an important regulator of PTH secretion and has both direct and indirect effects on PTH secretion. Indirect effects of calcitriol include an increase of intestinal calcium absorption and preventing skeletal resistance to PTH. Direct effects of calcitriol are decreased PTH gene transcription, an increase in parathyroid gland VDR expression, and restoring the elevated set-point for calcium toward normal.[4]

Skeletal Resistance to the Actions of Parathyroid Hormone

Skeletal resistance to the calcemic actions of PTH in CKD was first described in 1966 and it is thought to be an important factor in the development of SHPT. The pathogenesis of skeletal resistance is probably multifactorial.[12] It has been suggested that altered regulation of PTH receptors in bone may occur, resulting in downregulation or desensitization.[13] *In situ* hybridization studies of human bone have shown a downregulation of osteoblast PTH/PTHrP receptor mRNA in Stage 5 CKD, when compared to normal and non-uremic high turnover bone. This downregulation may represent the molecular basis for resistance of skeletal tissue to PTH in CKD.[12] Phosphorus retention and calcitriol deficiency are also known to be important factors in skeletal resistance to PTH.

Osteitis Fibrosa

Osteitis fibrosa is caused by SHPT and is the classic histological bone disorder in CKD that historically was the most common form of renal osteodystrophy. It is characterized by marrow fibrosis and an increased rate of bone turnover, including increases in both bone resorption and formation (see Chapter 3). The increased resorption is caused by an increase in the number and activity of osteoclasts. The increased bone formation is characterized by increases in osteoblasts and osteoid deposition. The osteoid is generally woven (nonlamellar) and thus abnormal.[1;14]

LOW-TURNOVER BONE DISEASE

Osteomalacia

Osteomalacia due to aluminum toxicity was a common form of bone disease in dialysis patients in the 1970s and 1980s. In the U.S., the incidence of osteomalacia is now quite low.[15] The primary source of aluminum accumulation in dialysis patients was first shown to be from water used to prepare the dialysate and subsequently from aluminum-based phosphate binders used to control hyperphosphatemia. Improved water purification standards and the discontinuation of aluminum-containing phosphate binders have markedly decreased the incidence of osteomalacia.[16;17] Although most cases of osteomalacia were due to aluminum, other factors may contribute to the development of osteomalacia, including vitamin D deficiency, metabolic acidosis, hypophosphatemia, and the trace elements, fluoride, and strontium.[17]

Osteomalacia develops because of inhibition of the mineralization process. The histological features are widened osteoid seams, an increase in the percentage of trabecular surface covered by osteoid, and a decreased bone formation rate. Cellular activity is low, with a paucity or absence of osteoblasts and osteoclasts. The low rate of osteoid deposition exceeds the low bone formation rate, resulting in osteoid accumulation.[1;17] Of interest is the relative PTH deficiency present in osteomalacia, which—at least in the aluminum-induced form— may be related to aluminum toxicity.

Aluminum-induced osteomalacia is associated with increased bone pain, muscle weakness, and bone fractures.[18] Other findings seen with aluminum toxicity include encephalopathy, microcytic anemia, and hypercalcemia.[19] Even though the incidence of aluminum-induced osteomalacia is decreasing, aluminum toxicity still occurs and should remain a diagnostic consideration. The K/DOQI Clinical Practice Guidelines on Bone Metabolism and Disease in CKD recommend that the source of aluminum should be identified and eliminated in all patients with plasma aluminum levels >60 µg/L, a positive DFO test, or clinical symptoms consistent with aluminum toxicity.[19] Aluminum toxicity is discussed in greater detail in Chapter 3

Adynamic Bone

Adynamic bone is characterized by a low number of osteoblasts, with the osteoclast number usually being normal or reduced. The sites of new bone formation are greatly reduced. Mineralization is decreased, but matches the decreased rate of osteoid deposition; thus osteoid thickness is normal. The reduction in osteoblast number and bone formation in adynamic bone may be a direct effect of a relative deficiency of PTH, although a number of other systemic inhibitory factors may also play a role.[17] In some cases of adynamic bone, osteoblast function improves over time, and the disorder can be considered reversible. In other cases, impairments in osteoblast activity persist, and bone formation and turnover cannot be restored to normal (Table 3).[20]

TABLE 3. CAUSES OF LOW-TURNOVER RENAL OSTEODYSTROPHY

Sustained	Reversible
Parathyroidectomy with low PTH levels	Calcitriol therapy
Steroid-induced osteopenia	Exogenous calcium loading
	-oral/dietary
	-dialysate
Osteoporosis	Immobilization
- estrogen deficiency	
-aging	
Diabetes mellitus	Aluminum toxicity

Abbreviation: PTH, parathyroid hormone.
Modified from: Salusky et al. J Am Soc Nephrol, Vol. 12, 2001.

Adynamic bone has become increasingly more common in CKD patients on maintenance dialysis and is especially prevalent in patients on continuous ambulatory peritoneal dialysis (CAPD). As many as 40% of adult patients on hemodialysis, and even more CAPD patients, have bone biopsy evidence of adynamic bone.[13] Risk factors for adynamic bone include diabetes mellitus, age, and aluminum accumulation, all of which have been associated with relatively low PTH levels. In some patients, the relative PTH deficiency may be a direct result of oversuppression from vitamin D and/or calcium supplementation.[14;20] In particular, rather than adynamic bone as a new entity, the idea has been advanced recently that it is simply a form of low bone turnover due to over-treatment of hyperparathyroidism with calcium binders and vitamin D, and consequent persistent positive calcium balance.[21]

Poor nutritional status may also be a significant factor in the development of adynamic bone.[22;23] At least in elderly dialysis patients, reduced protein and phosphorus intake and lower plasma phosphorus values correlate with lower PTH levels,[23] which, in turn, is probably a major factor in the development of adynamic bone.

Plasma calcium concentrations are often higher in patients with adynamic bone, due to a decreased capacity of the skeleton to buffer an exogenous calcium load from such sources as calcium-based phosphate binders or dialysate solutions.[20;24] A recent study of dialysis patients that compared bone histomorphometry characteristics to arterial calcification found that low bone activity/adynamic bone was associated with increased vascular calcification.[25] It has been reported that patients with adynamic bone have fewer musculoskeletal symptoms compared to patients with hyperparathyroid bone disease.[20] However, there is also some evidence that adynamic bone may contribute to skeletal fractures in patients on dialysis. In one study, the risk of vertebral fracture was 22% greater in those whose PTH values were in the lowest tertile.[26] In another study, the incidence of hip fractures was higher in patients with lower plasma PTH levels.[27]

Mixed Disease

Mixed ROD displays features of high-turnover and low-turnover bone disease. Thus, both features of osteitis fibrosa and osteomalacia are present. The osteomalacia is sometimes a result of aluminum accumulation, but other factors such as hypocalcemia and hypophosphatemia can also contribute to its development. Mixed disease has become less common as aluminum exposure in dialysis patients has decreased.[1]

CLINICAL MANIFESTATIONS

Bone disease in CKD is generally asymptomatic. Symptoms usually do not appear until late in the course of renal osteodystrophy and they are frequently nonspecific and often subtle. When symptoms appear, significant biochemical abnormalities and histological evidence of bone disease are generally present. However, the severity of symptoms often does not correlate with biochemical, radiological, or histological changes.[4]

Bone Pain

In the present era, with the decreased incidence of aluminum-induced bone disease, bone pain is not a common symptom of ROD. When present, bone pain is expressed as a general ache and can be diffuse or localized to the knee, ankle, or heel. The most severe bone pain occurs with aluminum-induced osteomalacia, in which localized bone tenderness and fractures are common.[4]

Myopathy and Muscle Weakness

Muscle weakness is typically limited to the proximal musculature and can be caused by SHPT, phosphorus depletion, aluminum toxicity, or low vitamin D levels. Plasma levels of muscle enzymes are usually normal and electromyographic abnormalities are either absent or nonspecific.[4]

Spontaneous Tendon Rupture

Spontaneous tendon rupture has been associated with severe SHPT. Rupture is most common in the quadriceps or triceps tendons, and in the extensor tendons of the fingers.[4]

Pruritus

Pruritus is a common symptom in patients with CKD, and is associated with high PTH levels, hypercalcemia, high calcium-phosphorus product and metastatic calcifications. If a patient is complaining of pruritus, an assessment of the extent of hyperparathyroidism and compliance with phosphate binders should be conducted. In patients with severe hyperparathyroidism and pruritus that is unresponsive to medical treatment, a subtotal parathyroidectomy may improve the pruritus.[4]

Metastatic and Extraskeletal Calcifications

Extraskeletal calcification, either metastatic or involving the vasculature, is commonly seen in dialysis patients. In the last few years, vascular calcification has been shown to be associated with poor outcomes in CKD patients, and therefore has become a major focus of investigation. Other sites of extraskeletal calcification in CKD patients include soft tissue and the aortic and mitral valves. The disorder termed calciphylaxis or calcific uremic arteriolopathy (CUA) results in skin necrosis with large ulcers and is primarily vascular-related. CUA is seen both in combination with osteitis fibrosa—as a consequense of increased release of calcium and phosphate from bone—and as a complication of adynamic bone disease, due to the inability to form new bone. A detailed review of the pathogenesis and clinical consequences of extraskeletal calcification is provided in Chapter 5.

Dialysis-Associated Amyloidosis

Dialysis-related amyloidosis is caused by a progressive accumulation of β2-microglobulin.[4] The clinical manifestations of amyloidosis typically do not appear until patients have been on dialysis for 8-12 years. Patients develop a disabling arthropathy due to amyloid deposits in articular and periarticular joints.

The clinical manifestations of amyloidosis in dialysis patients include carpal tunnel syndrome and joint swelling. The arthropathy is usually insidious and follows a progressive course. It usually manifests as arthralgias, frequently affecting the shoulder. Other clinical manifestations include chronic tenosynovitis of the finger flexors.[4]

X-ray examination may reveal subchondral bone cysts or erosions that increase in size and number over time, and appear to have a symmetrical distribution.[4] Biopsy and histological examination using Congo Red staining is the only definitive diagnostic technique for β2-microglobin amyloidosis.

CONCLUSIONS

Several studies have shown that bone changes develop early in the course of CKD. In one study, 84 patients with creatinine clearances <5 mL/min prior to the start of dialysis, underwent bone biopsies. Sixty-two percent of the patients had abnormal bone histology. The most common finding was adynamic bone disorder (23%), followed by mixed lesions (18%), osteomalacia (12%), and osteitis fibrosa (9%).[28] ROD was also common in a study of 176 CKD patients with a creatinine clearance between 15-50 mL/min. Abnormal bone histology was present in 75% of the patients. The mean creatinine clearance of these patients was 30.8 mL/min versus 35.9 mL/min in the 25% of patients with normal bone histology. The primary abnormality was osteitis fibrosa (55%), followed by mixed lesions (14%), adynamic bone (5%), and osteomalacia (1%).[29] Similar results were encountered in a study of 30 patients prior to being placed on dialysis. All of the patients had some form of bone histological abnormality. Fifty percent were diagnosed with osteitis fibrosa, 27% adynamic bone, 13% mixed lesions, and 7% osteomalacia.[15] Thus, it is important to recognize that nearly all patients with Stage 5 CKD will have some form of ROD, even though symptoms may rarely be experienced in the early stages of CKD.

REFERENCES

1. Hruska KA: Growth factors and cytokines in renal osteodystrophy, in Bushinsky DA (ed): Renal Osteodystrophy, Philadelphia, 1998, pp 221-255

2. Martinez I, Saracho R, Montenegro J, Llach F: A deficit of calcitriol synthesis may not be the initial factor in the pathogenesis of secondary hyperparathyroidism. Nephrol Dial Transplant 11 Suppl 3:22-28, 1996

*3. Felsenfeld AJ: Considerations for the treatment of secondary hyperparathyroidism in renal failure. J Am Soc Nephrol 8:993-1004, 1997

4. Martin KJ, Gonzalez EA, Slatopolsky EA: Renal osteodystrophy, in Brenner BM, Rector FC (eds): The Kidney, Philadelphia, 2004, pp 2256-2296

*5. Silver J, Kilav R, Naveh-Many T: Mechanisms of secondary hyperparathyroidism. Am J Physiol Renal Physiol 283:F367-F376, 2002

*6. Tallon S, Berdud I, Hernandez A, Concepcion MT, Almaden Y, Torres A, Martin-Malo A, Felsenfeld AJ, Aljama P, Rodriguez M: Relative effects of PTH and dietary phosphorus on calcitriol production in normal and azotemic rats. Kidney Int 49:1441-1446, 1996

7. Bover J, Jara A, Trinidad P, Rodriguez M, Martin-Malo A, Felsenfeld AJ: The calcemic response to PTH in the rat: effect of elevated PTH levels and uremia. Kidney Int 46:310-317, 1994

8. Slatopolsky E: The role of calcium, phosphorus and vitamin D metabolism in the development of secondary hyperparathyroidism. Nephrol Dial Transplant 13 Suppl 3:3-8, 1998

*9. Llach F, Bover J: Renal Osteodystrophies, in Brenner BM, Rector FC (eds): The Kidney, Philadelphia, 2000, pp 2103-2186

10. Fukuda N, Tanaka H, Tominaga Y, Fukagawa M, Kurokawa K, Seino Y: Decreased 1,25-dihydroxyvitamin D3 receptor density is associated with a more severe form of parathyroid hyperplasia in chronic uremic patients. J Clin Invest 92:1436-1443, 1993

*11. Kifor O, Moore FD, Jr., Wang P, Goldstein M, Vassilev P, Kifor I, Hebert SC, Brown EM: Reduced immunostaining for the extracellular Ca2+-sensing receptor in primary and uremic secondary hyperparathyroidism. J Clin Endocrinol Metab 81:1598-1606, 1996

12. Hoyland JA, Picton ML: Cellular mechanisms of renal osteodystrophy. Kidney Int Suppl 73:S8-13, 1999

13. Sherrard DJ, Hercz G, Pei Y, Maloney NA, Greenwood C, Manuel A, Saiphoo C, Fenton SS, Segre GV: The spectrum of bone disease in end-stage renal failure—an evolving disorder. Kidney Int 43:436-442, 1993

14. Hruska KA, Teitelbaum SL: Renal osteodystrophy. N Engl J Med 333:166-174, 1995

15. Hutchison AJ, Whitehouse RW, Boulton HF, Adams JE, Mawer EB, Freemont TJ, Gokal R: Correlation of bone histology with parathyroid hormone, vitamin D3, and radiology in end-stage renal disease. Kidney Int 44:1071-1077, 1993

16. Antonsen JE, Sherrard DJ: Renal osteodystrophy: past and present. Seminars in Dialysis 9:296-302, 1996

17. Couttenye MM, D'Haese PC, Verschoren WJ, Behets GJ, Schrooten I, De Broe ME: Low bone turnover in patients with renal failure. Kidney Int Suppl 73:S70-S76, 1999

18. Llach F: Renal bone disease. Transplant Proc 23:1818-1822, 1991

19. National Kidney Foundation: K/DOQI clinical practice guidelines for bone metabolism and disease in chronic kidney disease. Am J Kidney Dis 42: 4 Suppl 3:1-201, 2003

20. Salusky IB, Goodman WG: Adynamic renal osteodystrophy: is there a problem? J Am Soc Nephrol 12:1978-1985, 2001

21. Parfitt AM: Renal bone disease: a new conceptual framework for the interpretation of bone histomorphometry. Curr Opin Nephrol Hypertens 12:387-403, 2003

22. Fukagawa M, Akizawa T, Kurokawa K: Is aplastic osteodystrophy a disease of malnutrition? Curr Opin Nephrol Hypertens 9:363-367, 2000

*23. Lorenzo V, Martin M, Rufino M, Jimenez A, Malo AM, Sanchez E, Hernandez D, Rodriguez M, Torres A: Protein intake, control of serum phosphorus, and relatively low levels of parathyroid hormone in elderly hemodialysis patients. Am J Kidney Dis 37:1260-1266, 2001

24. Kurz P, Monier-Faugere MC, Bognar B, Werner E, Roth P, Vlachojannis J, Malluche HH: Evidence for abnormal calcium homeostasis in patients with adynamic bone disease. Kidney Int 46:855-861, 1994

*25. London GM, Marty C, Marchais SJ, Guerin AP, Metivier F, de Vernejoul MC: Arterial calcifications and bone histomorphometry in end-stage renal disease. J Am Soc Nephrol 15:1943-1951, 2004

26. Atsumi K, Kushida K, Yamazaki K, Shimizu S, Ohmura A, Inoue T: Risk factors for vertebral fractures in renal osteodystrophy. Am J Kidney Dis 33:287-293, 1999

27. Coco M, Rush H: Increased incidence of hip fractures in dialysis patients with low serum parathyroid hormone. Am J Kidney Dis 36:1115-1121, 2000

28. Spasovski GB, Bervoets AR, Behets GJ, Ivanovski N, Sikole A, Dams G, Couttenye MM, De Broe ME, D'Haese PC: Spectrum of renal bone disease in end-stage renal failure patients not yet on dialysis. Nephrol Dial Transplant 18:1159-1166, 2003

*29. Hamdy NA, Kanis JA, Beneton MN, Brown CB, Juttmann JR, Jordans JG, Josse S, Meyrier A, Lins RL, Fairey IT: Effect of alfacalcidol on natural course of renal bone disease in mild to moderate renal failure [see comments]. BMJ 310:358-363, 1995

*Suggested Reading

DIAGNOSIS OF BONE AND MINERAL DISORDERS

Kevin J. Martin

Masafumi Fukagawa

Hartmut H. Malluche

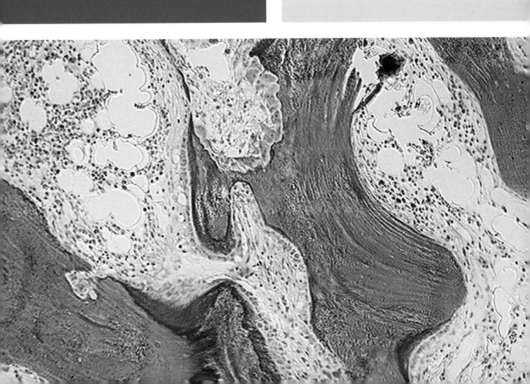

CHAPTER 3

DIAGNOSIS OF BONE AND MINERAL DISORDERS

Kevin J. Martin, Masafumi Fukagawa and Hartmut H. Malluche

The pathogenesis of renal bone disease or osteodystrophy (ROD) is complex and multifactorial. No single diagnostic procedure or test has sufficient specificity or reliability to accurately evaluate and determine a treatment regimen in the broad spectrum of bone disorders that develop in the course of chronic kidney disease (CKD). In order to successfully manage alterations in bone and mineral metabolism, multiple diagnostic parameters need to be considered and followed throughout the course of CKD.

The measurement and evaluation of several biochemical markers of bone and mineral metabolism are necessary for diagnosing and treating bone and mineral disorders in CKD. Evaluation of plasma calcium, phosphorus, parathyroid hormone (PTH), and total alkaline phosphatases are the core measurement standards (Tables 1 & 2). Additional markers of bone metabolism include plasma concentrations of bone-specific alkaline phosphatase, osteocalcin, and collagen breakdown products. Biomarkers provide valuable information in the overall assessment of ROD, yet no single marker is highly predictive of the underlying bone disease.

TABLE 1. MONITORING FREQUENCY AND TARGET RANGES FOR CALCIUM AND PHOSPHORUS FOR CKD STAGES[10]

CKD Stage	GFR range (mL/min/1.73m²)	Measurement frequency*	Total corrected plasma calcium	Plasma phosphorus	Calcium X Phos Product
3	30-59	Every 12 months	Normal range for laboratory	2.7-4.6 mg/dL (0.87-1.49 mmol/L)	<55 mg²/dL² (4.44 mmol²/L²)
4	15-29	Every 3 months	Normal range for laboratory	2.7-4.6 mg/dL (0.87-1.49 mmol/L)	<55 mg²/dL² (4.44 mmol²/L²)
5	<15	Every month	8.4-9.5 mg/dL (2.10-2.37 mmol/L)	3.5-5.5 mg/dL (1.13-1.78 mmol/L)	<55 mg²/dL² (4.44 mmol²/L²)

*Measurements should be made more frequently if the patient is receiving concomitant therapy for the abnormalities in the plasma levels of calcium, phosphorus, or PTH.

Abbreviations: CKD, chronic kidney disease; GFR, glomerular filtration rate.

TABLE 2. MONITORING FREQUENCY AND TARGET RANGES FOR PTH BY CKD STAGES[10]

CKD Stage	GFR range (mL/min/1.73m²)	Measurement frequency*	Total corrected plasma calcium	Intact PTH
3	30-59	Every 12 months	Normal range for laboratory	35-70 pg/mL (3.85-7.7 pmol/L)
4	15-29	Every 3 months	Normal range for laboratory	70-110 pg/mL (7.7-12.1 pmol/L)
5	<15	Every month	8.4-9.5 mg/dL (2.10-2.37 mmol/L)	150-300 pg/mL (16.5-33 pmol/L)

*Measurements should be made more frequently if the patient is receiving concomitant therapy for abnormalities in the plasma levels of PTH.

Abbreviations: CKD, chronic kidney disease; GFR, glomerular filtration rate.

Clinical signs and symptoms—such as bone pain, muscle weakness, pruritus, calcific uremic arteriolopathy, and fractures—appear late in the course of ROD and the severity of the symptoms does not always correlate well with the biochemical and bone histology abnormalities. Radiographic imaging can provide valuable information on the presence of severe bone abnormalities. However, it provides little information on the underlying pathogenic mechanisms.

When considered in combination and trended over time, clinical symptoms, radiographic imaging, and biomarkers can be used to successfully diagnose and treat the majority of CKD patients; however, to date, only the histological analysis of a bone biopsy can accurately determine the underlying bone abnormality.

BONE BIOPSY

Bone biopsy is the most powerful and informative diagnostic tool for determination of abnormalities in bone turnover. It is the gold standard to which all other biochemical and noninvasive assessments of bone metabolism must be compared. It does have the perceived disadvantage of being an invasive and potentially painful procedure that requires significant technical expertise to be correctly performed, analyzed, and interpreted.

The increased use of bone biopsy in research and as a clinical diagnostic tool has led to: improved instrumentation and biopsy techniques; rapid availability of results due to more well trained histomorphometrists; advances in sample processing techniques; and standardization of reporting nomenclature, allowing easier clinical interpretation of results.

Bone Biopsy Technique

An important prerequisite to enhance the value of a biopsy is labeling of the bone mineralization front at timed intervals. This procedure allows the addition of dynamic measures of bone turnover and rates of bone formation to static measures of bone structure, formation, and resorption.[1] It is accomplished by administering antibiotics from the tetracycline family that have an affinity for the surfaces of actively forming bone, and form complexes that have a spontaneous fluorescence. The best approach is a double-labeling technique that provides information on mineralization rate and bone formation.[2] This involves administration of tetracycline hydrochloride 500 mg BID for 2 days, followed by an 8- to 15-day interval without the antibiotic and then another 2- to 4-day course of demeclocycline hydrochloride 300 mg BID. The biopsy is then performed 4-6 days after the last dose of demeclocycline. A shorter labeling period with a single, larger oral tetracycline dose, followed by 6 days off, and then another single oral dose has also been used clinically.[3] Double labeling with the two different forms of tetracycline cogeners provides distinct colored fluorescence, making it easier to distinguish the labeled layers.

The site of choice for a bone biopsy is the anterior iliac crest. It is easily accessible and is minimally affected by local forces that can influence bone remodeling. Patients are typically given a mild sedative, such as intravenous midazolam, and then the biopsy site is infiltrated with local anesthetic. After positioning, draping, and surgical scrub, the specimen is obtained with a manual trocar or an electric drill. The specimen can be obtained using a vertical or horizontal approach. The horizontal transilial approach is the most common and provides information on both inner and outer cortical bone, although the sample size is limited by the thickness of the iliac bone. The vertical approach allows assessment of subcortical and deep cancellous bone. It also minimizes the risk of bleeding.

The retrieved specimen requires fixation to inhibit postmortem changes, followed by dehydration with ethanol. The specimen is then embedded in a plastic monomer and sectioned using a carbide- or diamond-edged microtome. Various staining techniques are available to assist in differentiating calcified and osteoid bone, or determining aluminum accumulation. There are several excellent references that describe bone biopsy and histomorphometry techniques in detail.[1;4-6]

Complications

In experienced hands, complications from bone biopsies are rare and include hematoma, pain, wound infection, and occasionally, neuropathy. In an analysis of 14,810 biopsies from 18 centers performing routine biopsies, the overall frequency of complications was 0.52%.[7] Patient reports of pain range from none to moderate, but rarely severe. In an assessment of pain experienced in 37 patients during and after biopsy, 21% reported no pain, 46% reported acceptable pain, 30% moderate pain and a single patient (3%) reported severe pain. This is consistent with other reports when local anesthesia is applied to the external and internal surfaces of the ilium.[8]

Histological Abnormalities of Bone in CKD

The alterations in bone metabolism associated with CKD can range from predominantly high-turnover bone disease (hyperparathyroid bone disease) to low-turnover bone disease or a mixed uremic osteodystrophy. Low-turnover conditions can include osteomalacia or adynamic bone. This classification of bone pathology is based on both static and dynamic parameters obtained from a bone biopsy with prior tetracycline labeling (see Table 3).

TABLE 3. CHANGES IN HISTOMORPHOMETRIC PARAMETERS WITH TYPE OF RENAL BONE DISEASE

Classification		Activation frequency (Year⁻¹)	Osteoblast surface/bone surface (%)	Fibrosis surface/bone surface (%)	Erosion surface/bone surface (%)	Mineralization lag time (days)	Osteoid thickness (μM)	Bone formation rate/bone surface (mm³/cm²/yr)
Normal Bone		0.49-0.72	2-5	0	3.7-5.0	<50	4-20	1.8-3.8
Hyperparathyroid Bone Disease	Moderate	0.49-3.0	2-20	1-20	1-10	<50		1.9-15.5
	Severe	>3.0	>20	>20	>10	<50		>15.5
Adynamic Bone Disease	With decrease in bone formation and bone erosion	<0.49	<5		<5			<1.8
	With decrease in bone formation and increase in bone erosion	<0.49	<5		>5			<1.8
Low-Turnover Osteomalacia		<0.49				>100	>20	<1.8
Mixed Renal Osteodystrophy	With prevailing Hyperparathyroid component	>0.72				>50		>3.8
	With prevailing mineralization defect	<0.72				>50	>20	<3.8

Parameters based on database from HH Malluche and MC Faugere, University of Kentucky-Lexington

Predominant hyperparathyroid bone disease

The primary histological feature of hyperparathyroid bone disease is a marked increase in bone turnover, both formation and resorption, with endosteal (peritrabecular) fibrosis. There are numerous abnormal remodeling sites with increased osteoblastic and osteoclastic activity. The extensive osteoblastic activity leads to excess unmineralized bone matrix (osteoid). Osteoid surface and volume increase, and the osteoid seam can thicken due to overproduction of collagen. There is a marked increase in the number of osteoclasts and resorption surface. Numerous dissecting resorption cavities can be seen where osteoclasts have tunneled into trabecules. The mineral apposition rate and the number and extent of mineralization sites are increased (Figure 1).

FIGURE 1. PREDOMINANT HYPERPARATHYROID BONE DISEASE

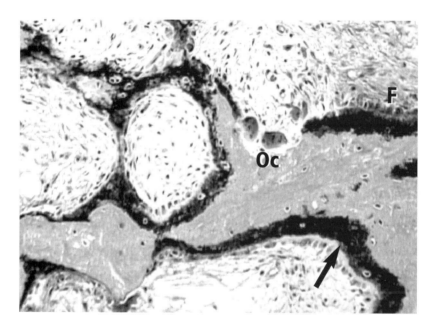

High fraction of trabecular surface covered by osteoid seams (arrow). High osteoid-osteoblast interface. High bone-osteoclast interface with appearance of deep resorption lacuna (Oc). Marrow fibrosis (F). Undecalcified, 3 μm thick section of human iliac bone (modified Masson-Goldner stain, 125 magnification). (From Malluche, H.H. et al., Kidney Int Suppl 73: S-21, 1999. Reprinted with permission.)

Low-turnover bone disease

Low-turnover disease, representing the other end of the ROD spectrum from hyperparathyroid bone disease, is characterized by a profound decrease in active remodeling sites. Few osteoblasts or osteoclasts are visible, and there is a predominance of lamellar bone structure with few active bone formation sites and markedly reduced mineralization surface. Low-turnover bone disease can be divided into two distinct subgroups: osteomalacia (OM) and adynamic bone disease (ABD).

OM is characterized by an accumulation of unmineralized bone matrix. The reduction in mineralization precedes (or is more pronounced than) the inhibition of collagen deposition (Figure 2). The unmineralized bone makes up a sizable portion of the trabecular bone volume. Lamellar osteoid volume is increased, with wide osteoid seams that cover much of the trabecular surface. No endosteal fibrosis is seen. Osteomalacia is frequently accompanied by an accumulation of aluminum in the bone.

FIGURE 2. LOW-TURNOVER OSTEOMALACIA

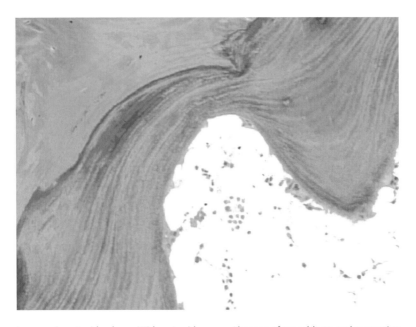

Increase in osteoid volume. Wide osteoid seams. Absence of osteoblasts and resorption surface. Undecalcified, 3 μm thick section of human iliac bone (modified Masson-Goldner stain, x 200 magnification). (From Malluche, H.H. et al., Kidney Int Suppl 73: S-21, 1999. Reprinted with permission.)

ABD is a primary defect in bone formation, accompanied by a parallel decrease in bone mineralization. Bone volume is frequently reduced. A primary differentiating feature of ABD is the absence of, or only a few, osteoid seams (Figure 3).

Decrease in bone cell activity is a dynamic phenomenon. Depending on where in the process this decline in bone formation and resorption is intersected by the biopsy, various degrees of changes in cellular activity can be seen. Generally, a decrease in osteoblastic activity precedes the decline in osteoclastic activity. Therefore, in many patients, one observes decreased osteoblasts with normal or even relatively high osteoclast numbers and activity, i.e., bone resorption exceeds formation. This negative balance leads to bone loss with reduced bone mineral density. However, in the later stages of low bone turnover, both osteoblast and osteoclast activity are equally suppressed.

FIGURE 3. ADYNAMIC BONE DISEASE

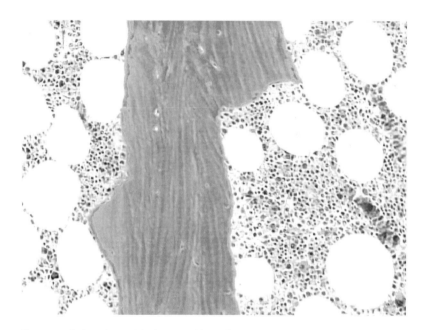

No accumulation of osteoid. Absence of bone formation. Absence of active bone resorption. Undecalcified, 3 μm thick section of human iliac bone (modified Masson-Goldner stain, x125 magnification). (From Malluche, H.H. et al., Kidney Int Suppl 73: S-21, 1999. Reprinted with permission.)

Mixed renal osteodystrophy

Mixed ROD is characterized by a combination of hyperparathyroid bone and defective mineralization. These features coexist in varying degrees in different patients. Bone volume/tissue volume is extremely variable depending on the predominant pathogenic cause. There is usually an increased number of remodeling sites and osteoclasts. Areas of high activity, bone cells, peritrabecular fibrosis, and woven osteoid seams coexist with areas of reduced activity (Figure 4).

FIGURE 4. MIXED UREMIC OSTEODYSTROPHY

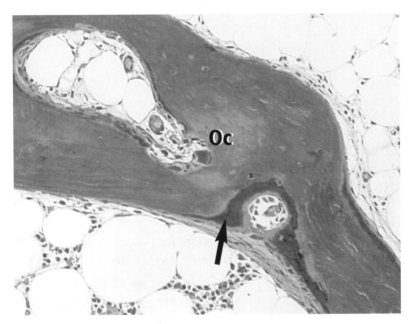

Increased fraction of trabecular surface covered by osteoid. Osteoid seams are wide or normal (arrow). Resorption lacunae with osteoclasts (Oc). Evidence of some peritrabecular fibrosis. Undecalcified, 3 μm thick section of human iliac bone (modified Masson-Goldner stain, x125 magnification. (From Malluche, H.H. et al., Kidney Int Suppl 73: S-21, 1999. Reprinted with permission.)

Indications for Bone Biopsy

In order to properly treat bone disease in CKD it is necessary to determine the patient's bone turnover status. Plasma PTH is an important parameter used to assess bone turnover in CKD Stage 5; however, its reliability—particularly when intact PTH levels are between 100 and 500 pg/mL—is inconsistent.[9] Bone biopsies provide an accurate depiction of bone metabolism, allowing a treatment approach tailored to the level of bone turnover and the degree of aluminum accumulation. If osteitis fibrosa (with elevated turnover rate) is the predominant histological finding, more aggressive therapy to reduce PTH (or a parathyroidectomy) may be indicated. In contrast, patients with bone histology indicating low-turnover disease in the presence of extensive aluminum deposits may be treated with a chelating agent. In the absence of aluminum accumulation, histological evidence of adynamic bone suggests that measures to increase PTH levels might be considered. A bone biopsy should be considered prior to a parathyroidectomy in any patient with previous aluminum exposure.

The K/DOQI Guidelines on Bone Metabolism and Disease in CKD recommend a bone biopsy be considered for Stage 5 CKD patients with the following conditions:[10]

- fractures with minimal or no trauma (pathological fractures);
- intact plasma PTH levels between 100-500 pg/mL (11.0-55.0 pmol/L) with coexisting conditions such as unexplained hypercalcemia, severe bone pain, or unexplained increases in bone alkaline phosphatase activity; or
- suspected aluminum bone disease, based upon clinical symptoms or history of aluminum exposure.

BIOCHEMICAL MARKERS OF BONE AND MINERAL METABOLISM

There are a number of biochemical parameters that can be measured to assist in the diagnosis and management of the bone and mineral abnormalities of CKD. They all have some limitations in diagnostic capacity. Ongoing studies on the correlation of specific biochemical parameters to actual bone metabolism, as demonstrated by bone biopsy, will enhance their clinical value. The usefulness of these biomarkers is enhanced when they are used to monitor trends over time, and when several are evaluated concomitantly.

Plasma Calcium

Calcium is present in blood in three forms: as ionized calcium (48%), bound to proteins (40%), and complexed with various anions, such as phosphate, citrate, and bicarbonate (12%).[11] Albumin is the predominant binding protein, accounting for approximately 90% of the calcium binding.

Total plasma calcium

In the clinical setting, total plasma calcium is the most common measurement of calcium status. While reference ranges vary between laboratories, normal values for total calcium in adults generally range from 8.4-10.2 mg/dL (2.1-2.6 mmol/L).* The normal range for total plasma calcium is slightly higher in children, particularly in those under 6 years of age. The amount of calcium bound to protein is dependent on plasma albumin concentration and pH.

Ionized calcium

Calcium, in its ionized form, is the fraction of blood calcium that is critical to physiological processes and is the best indicator of an individual's calcium status. It is technically more difficult to measure than total calcium; nevertheless, nearly all laboratories are now able to measure ionized calcium accurately. A normal reference range for ionized calcium concentrations is approximately 4.4-5.2 mg/dL (1.1-1.3 mmol/L), although this range may vary considerably depending on the laboratory assay technique.

* The molecular weight of calcium is 40.08 and its valence is 2. Calcium concentration expressed in mg/dL can be converted to mmol/L by dividing by 4, and to mEq/L by dividing by 2. (See Conversion Table in Appendix)

Corrected calcium

Total calcium levels are affected by the degree of protein binding. In situations where plasma albumin levels are abnormal, total calcium may not accurately reflect the patient's calcium status. In an effort to account for this inaccuracy in total calcium values, several formulas have been devised. One of the more commonly used formulas to provide a "corrected" calcium value is to add 0.8 mg/dL (0.2 mmol/L) to the measured total calcium for each 1.0 g/dL (10 g/L) decrease in albumin below 4.0 g/dL (40 g/L). Thus, a patient with a normal total calcium concentration of 10.0 mg/dL (2.5 mmol/L) and a plasma albumin level of 2.0 g/dL (20 g/L) would have a corrected calcium concentration of 11.6 mg/dL (2.9 mmol/L), indicating a significantly high plasma calcium level.[†] These corrections provide a better estimation of calcium status in some patients; however, they incorrectly predict calcium status in up to 30% of patients when correlated with actual ionized calcium levels.[12] Measurement of ionized calcium is preferable in the presence of altered plasma albumin concentration or plasma pH. The rationale for correcting a calcium measurement downwards in patients with albumin levels above 4 g/dL is questionable.

Plasma Phosphorus

The terms phosphorus concentration and phosphate concentration are often used interchangeably, although strictly speaking they should not be. While phosphorus is the chemical element in the body, it is never found in its free state, but occurs instead as phosphate ions (the most common of which are $H_2PO_4^-$, HPO_4^{2-}, and PO_4^{3-}). Phosphorus circulates in the plasma in the form of phosphate ions, which is the physiologically active form. Clinical assays for "phosphorus" typically measure phosphate ion concentration and the results are reported as elemental phosphorus concentrations.

Plasma phosphorus levels can vary significantly depending on the time of day and recent dietary phosphorus intake. It is not unusual to see a transient postprandial decrease in plasma phosphorus levels. For maximum accuracy, phosphorus levels should be evaluated with the patient fasting. Normal ranges for phosphorus are laboratory-specific, with the typical range of 2.5-4.5 mg/dL (0.8-1.44 mmol/L).[‡] It is critical that specimens are processed correctly, with prompt separation of red blood cells to minimize cell lysis that could result in falsely high levels.

Evaluation of calcium and phosphorus

Abnormalities in calcitriol production, kidney clearance, parathyroid function, and bone metabolism—along with some therapeutic interventions—result in significant alterations in calcium and phosphorus homeostasis in CKD. Abnormalities of calcium and phosphorus homeostasis appear to play a significant role in the morbidity and mortality associated with CKD. (See Chapter 4: Morbidity and Mortality.) The changes in mineral homeostasis begin early in the course of CKD Stage 3,[13;14] therefore evaluation and management throughout the progression of CKD is critical (Table 1).

[†] Corrected Calcuim = [(4.0-Measured Albumin) x 0.8 MG/DL] + Measured Total Calcium

[‡] The molecular weight of phosphorus is 30.98. Phosphorus concentration expressed in mg/dL can be converted to mmol/L by dividing by 3.1.

Parathyroid Hormone

Parathyroid hormone plays a critical role in the regulation of bone metabolism and mineral homeostasis and is the primary biomarker used in the evaluation of renal osteodystrophy. Plasma ionized calcium level is the primary regulator of PTH secretion from the parathyroid gland. Vitamin D and phosphorus levels also directly affect PTH synthesis and secretion.

The cascade of events in progressive CKD, decreased vitamin D production, hypocalcemia, and phosphorus retention lead to secondary hyperparathyroidism (SHPT), with associated high-turnover bone disease in many patients. Other patients with kidney failure develop low-turnover bone disease, termed adynamic bone disease, that is associated with relatively low levels of PTH. As the principal surrogate marker for bone histology, accurate measurement of PTH is critical for the diagnosis, monitoring, and treatment of the wide spectrum of skeletal disorders in CKD.

PTH metabolism

Biologically active PTH (1-84) is a polypeptide with an 84-amino-acid straight-chain sequence that is synthesized in and secreted from parathyroid cells. There are numerous factors that modulate PTH gene expression (production), PTH secretion, and parathyroid cell proliferation. Calcium concentration is the most significant determinant of minute-to-minute PTH secretion; however, vitamin D and phosphorus levels—together with calcium—are important in the regulation of PTH production and parathyroid cell proliferation.[15] The PTH (1-84) molecule readily undergoes metabolic degradation into smaller fragments within minutes. This breakdown begins within the parathyroid cells and is influenced by the ambient calcium concentration. Thus, when calcium levels are low, less breakdown occurs and more biologically active PTH (1-84) is released. When calcium is high, greater intracellular breakdown of PTH occurs. Both PTH fragments and the intact PTH (1-84) (iPTH) molecules are released from the parathyroid gland. Upon release, the iPTH molecule readily undergoes degradation by protease enzymes in the peripheral tissues, including the kidney and liver. §

PTH fragments in circulation generally are truncated at the amino terminus of the PTH molecule, and fragments such as PTH (37-84) and PTH (53-84) have been termed C-terminal fragments. Fragments with lesser truncations at the amino-terminal end of the PTH molecule such as PTH (7-84) have been termed N-terminally truncated PTH fragments. Various amounts of PTH peptides with an intact N-terminus may circulate in patients with CKD Stage 5 (Figure 5).

These PTH fragments have varying half-lives and biological activity on the PTH receptors. A PTH molecule with an intact amino terminus is required to interact with the classical PTH receptor, so iPTH or fragments with an intact N-terminus, such as PTH (1-34), have the greatest biological activity; however, they have a very short half-life. A primary mechanism for elimination of the PTH fragments is glomerular filtration and tubular degradation.[16] As a consequence, PTH fragments can accumulate in the presence of kidney failure or CKD Stage 5.

---

§ Because of the rapid breakdown and short half-life of the PTH molecule, proper specimen handling is critical to obtain accurate measurements. Several procedures, including rapid freezing of the plasma specimen or addition of EDTA to plasma to bind proteases have been developed to minimize degradation prior to assaying. It is essential to follow the assay manufacturers' guidelines to obtain valid results.

FIGURE 5. PARATHYROID HORMONE PEPTIDES

Circulating PTH Peptides

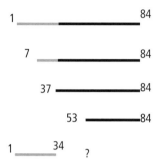

PTH peptides of varying structure are found in the serum. The 1-84 PTH molecule undergoes cleavage to smaller peptides both within the parathyroid gland before secretion and in the peripheral circulation. Each of fragments have varying degrees of intrinsic biologic activity. (From Martin, KJ and Gonzalez, E.A. Current Opinion in Nephrology & Hypertension. 10(5):569-574, 2001. Reprinted with permission.)

PTH Assays

The initial methodology used to measure PTH was a radioimmunoassay (RIA). Most of these original assays used antibodies that were directed towards the mid-or C-terminal region of PTH, and therefore measured both the iPTH molecule and C-terminal fragments. Because the C-terminal fragments accumulate in varying degrees in the plasma of patients with CKD, it was somewhat difficult to interpret the results obtained with the original assays.

To overcome this problem, immunometric assays were designed that used a two-antibody system. The first antibody (usually directed at the C-terminus) captured PTH from the sample. The captured PTH was then detected with a second, labeled antibody directed at the N-terminus. It was thought that these two-site assays would only detect the biologically active iPTH molecule. The result of the assay was referred to as iPTH to differentiate it from assays that measured both intact and truncated PTH molecules. These assays provided a more valid interpretation of parathyroid activity in kidney failure and have been the predominant assay used over the last decade. The iPTH assay has been used in the majority of recent therapeutic clinical trials, and it has been widely examined as a biomarker for bone metabolism. It is therefore currently the basis for most treatment protocols. The recommendations in the K/DOQI Guidelines on Bone Metabolism and Disease in CKD for the treatment of elevated PTH levels in CKD are based on the iPTH assay (Table 2).[10]

Recent studies have provided compelling evidence that the iPTH assays measure not only intact PTH (1-84) molecules, but also large, N-terminally-truncated PTH fragments, such as PTH (7-84).[17;18] This has led to the development of second-generation assays for PTH, designed with detection antibodies that are specific to the amino-terminus of the molecule (Figure 6).[19;20] These new assays that measure just the PTH (1-84) molecule are commonly referred to as either "whole" PTH, "bio-intact" PTH, or "bioactive" PTH by their manufacturers.

FIGURE 6. THE EVOLUTION OF ASSAYS FOR PARATHYROID HORMONE

Immunodetection of PTH Using Two Different 2 - Site Immunometric Assays

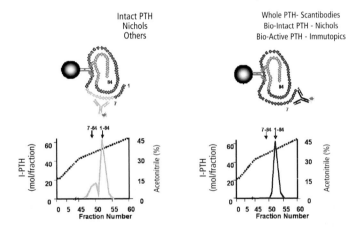

The "intact" PTH assay detects both the PTH (1-84) molecule and a major fragment PTH (7-84). The new generation PTH assays detect only the PTH (1-84) molecule. (Adapted from Martin, KJ and Gonzalez, E.A. Current Opinion in Nephrology & Hypertension. 10(5):569-574, 2001)

These second-generation immunometric PTH assays do not detect the 7-84 fragments, resulting in measured PTH concentrations approximately 40%-50% lower than values determined by the first-generation iPTH immunometric assay.[19;21;22] In general, results from the two types of assay have been shown to be highly correlated across a wide spectrum of PTH concentrations; however, the correlation is not consistent in some patients with CKD.[19;21-23] There is considerable variation in iPTH values among the manufacturers of the many iPTH assay kits. This variation may affect the usefulness of evaluating the ratio between PTH (1-84) and N-terminally truncated PTH fragments described below.[24]

It has been demonstrated that the large PTH (7-84) fragment may actually oppose the effects of PTH (1-84) on bone and contribute to the PTH resistance seen in CKD Stage 5, thereby potentially contributing to the development of adynamic bone disease.[22;25] By comparing the ratio of PTH (1-84) to this large C-terminal fragment in individual patients, it has been proposed that one may be able to more accurately depict bone turnover.[22;23] Other investigators have not been able to establish any correlation between this ratio and bone histology.[26] The clinical value of this ratio is currently under active investigation.

Interpretation of PTH values

In the general population, the normal range for iPTH is 10-65 pg/mL (1.1-7.15 pmol/L).**
These values coincide with normal bone turnover. In CKD, there is a progressive increase in skeletal resistance to PTH. The mechanism for this is not well understood, but is likely multifactorial, possibly related—at least in part—to downregulation of PTH receptors[27-29] and/or to the accumulation of inhibitory PTH fragments.[22] In the CKD Stage 5 population, normal bone turnover correlates better with plasma iPTH levels that are 2.5 to 4 times the upper limit of normal (150-300 pg/mL or 16.5-33 pmol/L)).[10] It is suggested, but without solid evidence, that in CKD Stage 3, optimal PTH levels are at the upper limit of normal and in CKD Stage 4, the optimal iPTH is between 70-110 pg/mL (7.7-12.1 pmol/L) (Table 2). Intact PTH levels are not highly specific for high-turnover bone disease, as a significant number of patients with CKD Stage 5 and iPTH levels between 150-450 pg/mL (16.5-49.5 pmol/L) have been found to have normal or low bone turnover, based on bone biopsy.[9;30] Similarly, a percentage of patients with iPTH levels <150 pg/mL (16.5 pmol/L) show histological evidence of high-turnover disease.[9;31] An iPTH level <65 pg/mL (7.15 pmol/L) in CKD Stage 5 is highly predictive of low-turnover bone disease. In dialysis patients with PTH levels between 100-500 pg/mL (11-55 pmol/L), an iliac crest bone biopsy with double tetracycline labeling and bone histomorphometric analysis is the only conclusive test to establish the type of bone turnover status and optimal therapeutic approach.

While PTH concentration is the primary clinical marker used in the assessment of bone turnover, there are other biochemical markers that may also be useful. The predictive power of PTH levels may be increased by concomitant consideration of these secondary markers. They can be divided into markers of bone formation or bone resorption.

MARKERS OF BONE FORMATION

Alkaline Phosphatase

Alkaline phosphatase (AP) is an isoenzyme that is produced primarily by the liver, and by osteoblasts in the skeletal system. The intestines, placenta, and kidneys also produce AP, although under normal conditions their contribution to total AP concentration is negligible. Therefore, in the absence of significant liver impairment, AP is a useful indicator of osteoblastic activity. Indeed, studies have indicated that elevated AP levels in uremia are primarily of skeletal origin and correlate with elevated PTH and histological changes indicative of high-turnover bone disease.[32-34]

Total AP levels, in conjunction with PTH, can be valuable in the differential diagnosis of high or low bone turnover. Patients with modest elevations in PTH (150-300 pg/mL, 16.5-33

** PTH levels expressed in pg/mL can be converted to pmol/L by multiplying by 0.11.

pmol/L) and normal AP levels are less likely to have significant elevations in bone turnover that require treatment. Serial measurements of AP in CKD patients can provide information on the progression of bone disease and the effectiveness of interventions to treat SHPT.[35] AP is typically not elevated in the presence of low-turnover bone disease,[36] although it is not exclusionary and may be elevated in some low-turnover bone states, particularly in the presence of aluminum toxicity[37] or osteomalacia.[4]

Measurement of total AP is common in the clinical setting, and therefore, is a convenient indicator of bone disease, although it lacks specificity. Patients with overt bone disease can have normal AP levels, and correlational studies between total AP measurements and bone histology have been inconsistent.[36;38;39] Liver abnormalities are common in dialysis patients. The potential contribution of liver dysfunction needs to be considered when evaluating AP levels. It is unlikely that the hepatic component of total AP will be significantly elevated in patients with normal values of hepatic enzymes.

Bone-specific alkaline phosphatase
Bone-specific alkaline phosphatase (BSAP) is the fraction of total AP that is specific to the osteoblast. In CKD patients, BSAP correlates well with iPTH levels and histomorphometric indices of SHPT,[30;40-42] and may be more accurate in predicting bone formation rates than iPTH, osteocalcin, or total AP.[40;42] When PTH and BSAP were used concurrently to evaluate bone disease, they had a positive predictive value of 96.7% for high-turnover disease (hyperparathyroid and mixed osteodystrophy combined) and 72.7% for low-turnover disease.[30] In comparison, when PTH and total AP were evaluated concurrently, the predictive values were 96.3% and 57.2%, respectively. In another histological analysis of patients on hemodialysis, plasma BSAP levels of 27 U/L or less were found to be a good index of adynamic bone disease, with a sensitivity and specificity of 78% and 86%, respectively.[43]

Osteocalcin
Osteocalcin (bone Gla-protein) is a noncollagenous protein that is present in bone matrix and is produced by osteoblasts.[44] Although its physiological role is not well understood, it appears to play an important role in bone formation.[45] It is generally thought that osteocalcin stimulates bone formation, but a study of osteocalcin-deficient mice showed an augmentation of bone formation and bone density—not a decrease, as might be expected.[46] The value of osteocalcin as a marker in CKD is complicated by its dependence on kidney filtration for excretion, resulting in accumulation of osteocalcin fragments in the plasma in patients with CKD Stage 5. There appears to be a fair amount of variability in the ability of the current assays to detect the various fragments.[47] Studies evaluating the correlation of osteocalcin levels with parameters of bone histology have been mixed. Some investigators have found that it correlates well, albeit weaker than PTH and BSAP,[32;42;48] while others have found a significant correlation.[30;49] In a study evaluating a newer assay methodology, reported to detect only intact osteocalcin, plasma osteocalcin levels were a good predictor of adynamic bone in dialysis patients with iPTH levels between 65-455 pg/mL (7.15-50.1 pmol/L).[50]

Procollagen type 1 carboxy-terminal extension peptides (PICP)
The major component of extracellular bone matrix is Type 1 collagen. Osteoblasts stimulate collagen formation through the intracellular production of procollagen. Measurement of C-terminal fragments of the procollagen peptide molecule (PICP) that are excised prior to the formation of osteoid fibrils can be used as an index for the rate of collagen synthesis and osteoblastic activity.[51] PICP levels are significantly correlated with biochemical and histological parameters of bone formation in CKD patients.[51;52] However, PICP levels correlate inversely to the fall in GFR.[41]

Markers of Bone Resorption

Collagen breakdown products
As collagen molecules in bone matrix are metabolized, byproducts are released into the circulation and are normally secreted in the urine. With impaired kidney function, these byproducts accumulate in the plasma.[41] As bone resorption increases, the breakdown of collagen increases; therefore, measurement of collagen breakdown products can provide a valuable indicator of bone resorption.

Pyridinoline (PYD) and deoxypyridinoline (DPD) are two of these bone collagen breakdown products that can be accurately measured and have been thoroughly studied.[47] Clinical studies in the dialysis population found a strong correlation between plasma PYD and DPD levels and levels of iPTH, BSAP, and bone histology.[48;53]

Procollagen Type 1 cross-linked carboxy-terminal telopeptide (ICTP) is another collagen derivative that is released during bone resorption. Studies to date have failed to show a good correlation between ICTP and other markers of resorption in patients with SHPT.[48;54]

Tartrate-resistant acid phosphatase
The osteoclast-specific portion of tartrate-resistant acid phosphatase, TRAP 5b, has recently been identified.[55] This acid phosphatase lysosomal enzyme is synthesized by osteoclasts, released into the circulation, and may be a good noninvasive marker of bone resorption. Some early clinical studies have found that plasma levels of TRAP 5b correlate well with iPTH levels in dialysis patients.[56]

General Remarks on Bone Biomarker Evaluation
The majority of studies on bone biomarkers evaluate the correlation of the marker to bone histology or other noninvasive markers. Correlational studies of this type provide information only on the relationship between the parameters, i.e., whether they occur in parallel, if they are proportional, etc. It is important to note that general correlations between bone markers and bone histology are not of great value in establishing underlying pathology, except between PTH and bone histomorphometry in severe SHPT (PTH levels > 600 pg/mL). For diagnostic purposes, it is critical to establish the sensitivity (proportion of people without the underlying pathology who have a negative test) and specificity (proportion of people with the underlying pathology who have a positive test result) of the marker.

Aluminum

Aluminum clearance is dependent on kidney excretion, so any intake of aluminum in CKD (Stages 4 and 5) can lead to its accumulation in tissues, including bone, brain, parathyroid, and other organs.[57] Clinical symptoms of aluminum toxicity can be neurological—such as altered consciousness, dementia, seizures, and speech abnormalities; or musculoskeletal—such as bone pain, proximal muscle weakness, and fractures. Other symptoms include microcytic anemia, without evidence of iron deficiency, and hypercalcemia in the absence of severe SHPT or vitamin D therapy.[10]

Aluminum-related bone disease and toxicity has become increasingly rare with the reduction in use of aluminum-based phosphate binders and the introduction of dialysis water treatment installations that remove aluminum. However, aluminum-based phosphate binders are still being used in some patients; therefore, aluminum toxicity remains a diagnostic consideration. The K/DOQI Guidelines on Bone Metabolism and Disease in CKD recommend that plasma aluminum levels be evaluated in all dialysis patients yearly and every 3 months in those receiving aluminum-containing medications.[10]

Plasma aluminum

Baseline plasma aluminum levels should be <20 µg/L.[10] In general, plasma aluminum levels reflect recent aluminum load and potential for accumulation, not necessarily overt toxicity. However, in the hemodialysis population, aluminum values >60 µg/L have a sensitivity of 82%, specificity of 86%, and a predictive value of 76% for the diagnosis of aluminum-related bone disease.[58] It has been recommended that a deferoxamine (DFO) test be performed on patients who have a plasma aluminum concentration between 60-200 µg/L with clinical symptoms of aluminum toxicity or those being considered for parathyroid surgery.[10]

Deferoxamine test

DFO is a chelating agent which can mobilize accumulated aluminum from the tissue stores into the plasma. The increment in plasma aluminum concentration after DFO infusion may be a good indicator of the risk of aluminum-related bone disease.[59] The test is accomplished by administering 5 mg/kg of DFO during the last hour of the dialysis session, with plasma aluminum measured before DFO infusion and 2 days later, before the next dialysis session.[10] Patients who have an increment in plasma aluminum of 50 µg/L or greater are likely to have aluminum-related bone disease; however, there are number of patients who will have increases in aluminum without histological evidence of bone accumulation. There are also a high number of false negatives with this test, so a smaller increment does not exclude aluminum toxicity.[60] To avoid acute aluminum toxicity, DFO testing should not be done if the baseline aluminum level is >200 µg/L. A positive DFO test, accompanied by PTH levels of <150 pg/mL, is predictive of aluminum-related bone disease.[10] Bone biopsy with aluminum staining is the only definitive diagnostic method.

β_2-microglobulin

β_2-microglobulin (β_2M) is a polypeptide that is involved in the lymphocyte-mediated immune response. It is a major constituent of the amyloid protein accumulation found in β_2-microglobulin amyloidosis (β_2MA; also called dialysis-related amyloidosis [DRA]) that is a frequent and disabling complication of long-term dialysis.[61;62] The kidney is the primary site for β_2M catabolism and excretion.[63] The normal reference range for plasma β_2M levels is 1.5-3.0 mg/L, but plasma levels are often 15-30 times higher in dialysis patients. Retention and accumulation of this type of amyloid protein is presumed to be the main pathogenic process underlying β_2MA. The accumulation occurs progressively, and clinical symptoms rarely appear in the first 5 years of dialysis.[64] The incidence of β_2MA increases progressively with dialysis duration, such that the majority of patients have clinical manifestations of β_2MA after 15 years of dialysis.[10]

The amyloid fibrils tend to deposit in tendons, in periarticular structures, at the ends of long bones and in the intervertebral disks.[62] The most common clinical manifestations include joint pain (particularly shoulder), hemarthrosis, carpal tunnel syndrome, flexor tenosynovitis in the hands, and destructive arthropathies and spondyloarthropathies,.[65;66] Carpal tunnel syndrome is the most prevalent—and usually the first—symptom of β_2MA.

Diagnosis

Radiographs, scintigraphy, ultrasound, and MRI can all provide information related to clinical manifestation of β_2MA, although none has been shown to be a reliable screening tool for β_2MA in dialysis. Plasma β_2M levels are elevated in most dialysis patients and do not correlate with clinical manifestations; therefore, they also have no value as a screening tool. The only definitive diagnostic technique is a biopsy demonstrating positive Congo Red staining and immunohistochemistry for the presence of β_2-microglobulin.[10]

Treatment

Other than kidney transplantation, there are no currently available therapies to stop the progression of β_2MA. Using high-flux biocompatible polyacrylonitrile and polysulfone dialysis membranes enhances β_2MA removal during hemodialysis and hemofiltration, and may slow the progression of β_2MA.[10;67] Medical therapy is limited to symptomatic approaches in ameliorating joint pain and inflammation.

DIAGNOSTIC IMAGING

Parathyroid Gland Imaging

Parathyroid imaging is commonly used to assist in identification and anatomical localization of the parathyroid glands (PTGs) prior to parathyroidectomy (PTX). In addition, it may provide valuable clinical information on the severity of SHPT, the responsiveness to medical therapy, and the need for surgical intervention.[68] There are several noninvasive imaging methods available to evaluate the PTGs, including ultrasonography, computed tomography (CT), magnetic resonance imaging (MRI), and scintigraphy.

The PTGs are most commonly present as a group of four; although between two and six glands are possible. They are usually divided into superior and inferior pairs located on the posterior surface of the thyroid gland. However, when the glands form during embryogenesis, they can migrate to locations varying from the upper neck to the mediastinum. To accommodate the increased demand for PTH production that occurs with SHPT, the parathyroid cells initially enlarge with general hypertrophy of the gland. As SHPT progresses, parathyroid cells proliferate and diffuse hyperplasia develops. If left unchecked, the proliferating cells often form nodules of abnormal tissue.[69] The cells within the nodular growth areas have a lower density of vitamin D and calcium-sensing receptors and therefore become less responsive to medical therapy.[70;71] (For a more detailed description of this process, see Chapter 4.) The ability to quantify the amount of nodular growth through PTG imaging should provide important clinical data to manage SHPT.

Serial imaging during treatment with calcitriol has been used to determine the degree of PTG suppression and efficacy of therapy for hyperparathyroidism. It was demonstrated that patients with at least one PTG >0.5 cm^3 (or 1.0 cm in diameter), as determined by ultrasonography, were more likely to be refractory to pulse calcitriol therapy.[72] Patients with enlargement of three or more glands with evidence of nodular hyperplasia and resistance to medical therapy have been considered as good candidates for PTX before the advent of cinacalcet treatment.[73;74]

PTG imaging can be used prior to surgical PTX, to pinpoint the location of the PTGs and identify any possible supernumerary or ectopic glands. This imaging may be particularly helpful in cases where re-exploration is required, or for recurrent hyperparathyroidism. It also provides information on which gland or tissue has the least nodular hyperplasia so that it can be harvested for autotransplantation. There is a higher risk of recurrence if tissue from nodular glands is used for PTG autografting.[75]

Parathyroid imaging techniques

Ultrasonography is used in the evaluation of the PTGs (Figure 7). It is noninvasive and, in experienced hands, appears to have sufficient specificity to accurately assess the extent and type of PTG hyperplasia. The quality of the information provided can be enhanced by incorporating Doppler color imaging to determine blood vessel density and blood flow velocity in the tissue.[76] Ultrasonography is also used for localization of parathyroid tissue when performing therapeutic percutaneous injection of the PTGs with ethanol or calcitriol.[77] This treatment modality is widely applied at present in Japan, but not in other countries.

Scintigraphy imaging uses radioisotope labeled proteins, most commonly 99-technetium-sestamibi, that are readily taken up by the overactive parathyroid cells. Scintigraphy has become a common method of presurgical localization of the PTG, although it appears to have a variable sensitivity and is of limited value for localizing all PTGs in SHPT.[78;79] The sensitivity of a sestamibi scan is greater when trying to localize a single gland in patients with recurrent SHPT.[79] MRI and CT scans sometimes can also provide valuable information on abnormal PTG localizations.[80]

FIGURE 7. ULTRASONOGRAPHY OF PARATHYROID GLAND

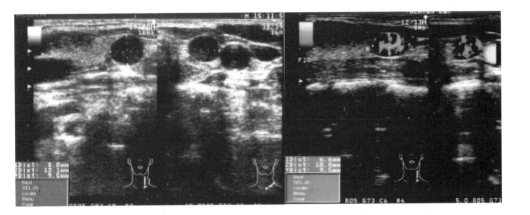

A. B-mode, B. Power Doppler flow mapping Volume of the gland is calculated by measuring three dimensions.(1) Positive blood flow within the gland highly suggests nodular hyperplasia. (B) arrowhead: parathyroid, CA: common carotid artery

PLAIN RADIOGRAPHS

In general, X-ray examination of bone provides limited information on renal osteodystrophy, primarily because pathological features are nonspecific and appear late in the course of the disease. Bone demineralization needs to be quite severe before it is detectable by X-ray.

The most common radiological feature of SHPT is subperiosteal erosions, which typically appear first on the radial surfaces of the middle phalanges.[81] Other sites that commonly show subperiosteal erosions include the upper end of the tibia, the necks of the femur and humerus, the lower ends of the radius and ulna, and the distal ends of the clavicle. These erosions can remain long after a change in the underlying metabolism of the bone; therefore, they have limited diagnostic value.[4] Looser zones (pseudofractures) are radiolucent areas occurring at right angles to the cortex and extending across a portion of the bone diameter. They are typically seen with osteomalacia, but they may also occur in patients with osteoporosis.[4]

Radiographic evidence suggests that β_2-microglobulin accumulation frequently is present prior to the onset of symptoms. Periarticular cystic bone lesions located in carpel or tarsal bone, the femoral or humeral head, distal radius, acetabulum, pubic symphysis, or tibial plateau is highly suggestive of dialysis-related amyloidosis.[81] Radiographs can also provide valuable information on extraskeletal calcification (Chapter 4).

BONE MINERAL DENSITY

Bone mineral density (BMD) is most commonly measured by dual-energy x-ray absorptiometry (DXA). DXA measures the mineral content/density of bone and is well established as a rapid, accurate, and noninvasive procedure to identify osteopenia/osteoporosis. Common sites of measurement include the proximal femur, radius, heel, and lateral or AP spine. BMD varies between sites; when evaluating risk factors, it must be compared to the site-specific standards. BMD measurements are a strong predictor of fracture risk in the general population and often are used to assess the efficacy of therapeutic interventions,[82;83] but they do not achieve the same degree of reliable information as the evaluation of changes in fracture rate does.

Reduced BMD is a common finding in dialysis patients,[84] who have a much greater risk of hip fracture than the general population.[85;86] BMD has been shown to correlate with biomarkers of high-turnover bone disease in CKD Stage 3 and 4 patients.[41]

However, the value of DXA in assessment of bone in CKD is not as clear. DXA does not provide specific information on bone turnover and quality, which is significantly altered in CKD. It does not correlate well with bone histology and provides no indication of the primary type of renal osteodystrophy—information that is critical in developing a treatment regimen.

Findings on the correlation of BMD measurements to fracture risk in the CKD population are inconsistent. Several studies have demonstrated a positive correlation between BMD and fractures,[87;88] although there appears to be a poor correlation with fracture rates when BMD is measured by lumbar spine DXA. BMD in CKD patients with vertebral and fragility fractures was similar to CKD patients without fractures.[89;90] These conflicting findings may be related to the site and technique used. Spinal BMD measurement might be affected by aortic calcifications frequently observed in CKD patients. In addition, trabecular bone sclerosis can occur with SHPT, resulting in an increased vertebral BMD despite disruption of structural integrity.[91] This is supported by the finding that, in CKD patients, BMD measurements of the cortical bone in the radius correlated better with fracture rates than lumbar spine BMD.[90] Measurement of BMD at the hip and radius may give better precision with fewer artifacts. Further studies in the CKD population are needed to determine the optimum sites for DXA measurement.

Quantitative Computed Tomography (qCT) is another procedure that can accurately measure BMD. It has distinct advantages over DXA in that it provides a three-dimensional image, unaffected by surrounding structures, allowing accurate measurement of bone dimensions and discernment of cortical versus trabecular bone. This is particularly advantageous with renal bone disease, where hyperparathyroidism can lead to sclerotic thickening of trabecular bone with increased BMD, while simultaneously stimulating resorption in cortical bone with significant reductions in BMD. In contrast, low-turnover bone disorders typically result in reductions in trabecular BMD.[92]

Following serial BMD measurements may provide valuable information on the progress of a patient's skeletal demineralization, but this should not be considered a diagnosis in itself or an independent indicator to determine the treatment regimen. BMD should be considered in combination with clinical assessment, bone and mineral biomarkers, and bone histology, when available.

CONCLUSIONS

The broad spectrum of underlying causes for the alterations in bone and mineral metabolism that accompany CKD provides a significant diagnostic challenge for the clinician. This diversity of pathophysiological mechanisms also means that a thorough, ongoing evaluation is critical in selecting the correct treatment course to minimize the morbidity and mortality that accompany these disorders. PTH has been widely used as a surrogate marker of bone metabolism, but recent studies have questioned its sensitivity and specificity as a marker for bone turnover. The newer PTH assays may enhance its diagnostic value. Evaluation of other biomarkers of bone metabolism may improve diagnostic accuracy. However, additional studies based on bone histomorphometry are clearly needed to evaluate the clinical value of these biomarkers of bone metabolism in CKD. Bone biopsy remains the best indicator of the underlying bone pathology, although its routine clinical use has been inhibited by the perceived disadvantages of accessibility, cost, and patient discomfort. Even if bone histology results are available, they must be considered within the context of the patient's vitamin D levels, parathyroid function, calcium and phosphorus balance, and risk factors for soft-tissue calcification and bone fracture when determining an individual treatment regimen.

REFERENCES

*1. Malluche HH, Monier-Faugere MC: The role of bone biopsy in the management of patients with renal osteodystrophy. J Am Soc Nephrol 4:1631-1642, 1994

2. Frost HM: Tetracycline-based histological analysis of bone remodeling. Calcif Tissue Res 3:211-237, 1969

3. Sherrard DJ, Maloney NA: Single-dose tetracycline labeling for bone histomorphometry. Am J Clin Pathol 91:682-687, 1989

4. Malluche HH, Faugere M: Atlas of Mineralized Bone Histology. New York, Karger, 1986,

5. Monier-Faugere MC, Langub MC, Malluche HH: Mineralized bone histology in normal and uremic states, in Bushinsky DA (ed): Renal Osteodystrophy, chap 3. Philadelphia, 1998, pp 49-87

*6. Monier-Faugere MC, Langub MC, Malluche HH: Bone Biopsoes: a modern approach, in Avioli LV, Krane SM (eds): Metabolic Bone Disease and Clinical Related Disorders, chap 8. San Diego, 1998, pp 237-273

7. Duncan H, Rao SD, Parfitt AM: Complications of bone biopsies, in Jee W, Parfitt A (eds): Bone Histomorphometry, Paris, 1981,

8. Johnson KA, Kelly PJ, Jowsey J: Percutaneous biopsy of the iliac crest. Clin Orthop 34-36, 1977

*9. Qi Q, Monier-Faugere MC, Geng Z, Malluche HH: Predictive value of serum parathyroid hormone levels for bone turnover in patients on chronic maintenance dialysis. Am J Kidney Dis 26:622-631, 1995

10. National Kidney Foundation: K/DOQI clinical practice guidelines for bone metabolism and disease in chronic kidney disease. Am J Kidney Dis 42:1-201, 2003

11. Moore EW: Ionized calcium in normal serum, ultrafiltrates, and whole blood determined by ion-exchange electrodes. J Clin Invest 49:318-334, 1970

12. Ladenson JH, Lewis JW, Boyd JC: Failure of total calcium corrected for protein, albumin, and pH to correctly assess free calcium status. J Clin Endocrinol Metab 46:986-993, 1978

13. Malluche HH, Ritz E, Lange HP, Kutschera L, Hodgson M, Seiffert U, Schoeppe W: Bone histology in incipient and advanced renal failure. Kidney Int 9:355-362, 1976

14. Ritz E, Krempien B, Mehls O, Malluche H: Skeletal abnormalities in chronic renal insufficiency before and during maintenance hemodialysis. Kidney Int 4:116-127, 1973

15. Silver J, Kronenberg HM: Parathyroid hormone: molecular biology and regulation, in Bilezikian JP, Raisz LG, Rodan GA (eds): Priniciples of bone biology, chap 24. New York, 1996, pp 325-346

16. Martin KJ, Hruska KA, Lewis J, Anderson C, Slatopolsky E: The renal handling of parathyroid hormone. Role of peritubular uptake and glomerular filtration. J Clin Invest 60:808-814, 1977

17. Brossard JH, Cloutier M, Roy L, Lepage R, Gascon-Barre M, D'Amour P: Accumulation of a non-(1-84) molecular form of parathyroid hormone (PTH) detected by intact PTH assay in renal failure: importance in the interpretation of PTH values. J Clin Endocrinol Metab 81:3923-3929, 1996

*18. Lepage R, Roy L, Brossard JH, Rousseau L, Dorais C, Lazure C, D'Amour P: A non-(1-84) circulating parathyroid hormone (PTH) fragment interferes significantly with intact PTH commercial assay measurements in uremic samples. Clin Chem 44:805-809, 1998

19. John MR, Goodman WG, Gao P, Cantor TL, Salusky IB, Juppner H: A novel immunoradiometric assay detects full-length human PTH but not amino-terminally truncated fragments: implications for PTH measurements in renal failure. J Clin Endocrinol Metab 84:4287-4290, 1999

*20. Martin KJ, Akhtar I, Gonzalez EA: Parathyroid hormone: new assays, new receptors. Semin Nephrol 24:3-9, 2004

21. Gao P, Scheibel S, D'Amour P, John MR, Rao SD, Schmidt-Gayk H, Cantor TL: Development of a novel immunoradiometric assay exclusively for biologically active whole parathyroid hormone 1-84: implications for improvement of accurate assessment of parathyroid function. J Bone Miner Res 16:605-614, 2001

*22. Slatopolsky E, Finch J, Clay P, Martin D, Sicard G, Singer G, Gao P, Cantor T, Dusso A: A novel mechanism for skeletal resistance in uremia. Kidney Int 58:753-761, 2000

23. Monier-Faugere MC, Geng Z, Mawad H, Friedler RM, Gao P, Cantor TL, Malluche HH: Improved assessment of bone turnover by the PTH-(1-84)/large C-PTH fragments ratio in ESRD patients. Kidney Int 60:1460-1468, 2001

24. Koller H, Zitt E, Staudacher G, Neyer U, Mayer G, Rosenkranz AR: Variable parathyroid hormone(1-84)/carboxylterminal PTH ratios detected by 4 novel parathyroid hormone assays. Clin Nephrol 61:337-343, 2004

25. Langub MC, Monier-Faugere MC, Wang G, Williams JP, Koszewski NJ, Malluche HH: Administration of PTH-(7-84) antagonizes the effects of PTH-(1-84) on bone in rats with moderate renal failure. Endocrinology 144:1135-1138, 2003

26. Coen G, Bonucci E, Ballanti P, Balducci A, Calabria S, Nicolai GA, Fischer MS, Lifrieri F, Manni M, Morosetti M, Moscaritolo E, Sardella D: PTH 1-84 and PTH "7-84" in the noninvasive diagnosis of renal bone disease. Am J Kidney Dis 40:348-354, 2002

27. Fournier A, Moriniere P, Cohen Solal ME, Boudailliez B, Achard JM, Marie A, Sebert JL: Adynamic bone disease in uremia: may it be idiopathicα Is it an actual disease? Nephron 58:1-12, 1991

28. Tian J, Smogorzewski M, Kedes L, Massry SG: PTH-PTHrP receptor mRNA is downregulated in chronic renal failure. Am J Nephrol 14:41-46, 1994

29. Urena P, Kubrusly M, Mannstadt M, Hruby M, Trinh MM, Silve C, Lacour B, Abou-Samra AB, Segre GV, Drueke T: The renal PTH/PTHrP receptor is down-regulated in rats with chronic renal failure. Kidney Int 45:605-611, 1994

30. Coen G, Ballanti P, Bonucci E, Calabria S, Centorrino M, Fassino V, Manni M, Mantella D, Mazzaferro S, Napoletano I, Sardella D, Taggi F: Bone markers in the diagnosis of low turnover osteodystrophy in haemodialysis patients. Nephrol Dial Transplant 13:2294-2302, 1998

31. Wang M, Hercz G, Sherrard DJ, Maloney NA, Segre GV, Pei Y: Relationship between intact 1-84 parathyroid hormone and bone histomorphometric parameters in dialysis patients without aluminum toxicity. Am J Kidney Dis 26:836-844, 1995

32. Canavese C, Barolo S, Gurioli L, Cadario A, Portigliatti M, Isaia G, Thea A, Marangella M, Bongiorno P, Cavagnino A, Peona C, Boero R, D'Amicone M, Cardelli R, Rossi P, Piccoli G: Correlations between bone histopathology and serum biochemistry in uremic patients on chronic hemodialysis. Int J Artif Organs 21:443-450, 1998

33. Hruska KA, Teitelbaum SL, Kopelman R: The predictability of the histologic features of uremic bone disease by noninvasive techniques. Metab Bone Dis Rel Res39-57, 1978

34. Pierides AM, Skillen AW, Ellis HA: Serum alkaline phosphatase in azotemic and hemodialysis osteodystrophy: a study of isoenzyme patterns, their correlation with bone histology, and their changes in response to treatment with 1alphaOHD3 and 1,25(OH)2D3. J Lab Clin Med 93:899-909, 1979

35. Cannella G, Bonucci E, Rolla D, Ballanti P, Moriero E, De Grandi R, Augeri C, Claudiani F, Di Maio G: Evidence of healing of secondary hyperparathyroidism in chronically hemodialyzed uremic patients treated with long-term intravenous calcitriol. Kidney Int 46:1124-1132, 1994

36. Llach F, Felsenfeld AJ, Coleman MD, Keveney JJ, Jr., Pederson JA, Medlock TR: The natural course of dialysis osteomalacia. Kidney Int Suppl 18:S74-S79, 1986

37. Hodsman AB, Sherrard DJ, Wong EG, Brickman AS, Lee DB, Alfrey AC, Singer FR, Norman AW, Coburn JW: Vitamin-D-resistant osteomalacia in hemodialysis patients lacking secondary hyperparathyroidism. Ann Intern Med 94:629-637, 1981

38. Malluche HH, Arnala I, Faugere MC: Values of noninvasive techniques in predicting bone histology. Ann Chir Gynaecol 77:246-250, 1988

39. Siede WH, Seiffert UB, Bundschuh F, Malluche HH, Schoeppe W: Alkaline phosphatase bone isoenzyme activity in serum in various degrees of micromorphometrically assessed renal osteopathy. Clin Nephrol 13:277-281, 1980

40. Jarava C, Armas JR, Salgueira M, Palma A: Bone alkaline phosphatase isoenzyme in renal osteodystrophy. Nephrol Dial Transplant 11 Suppl 3:43-46, 1996

*41. Rix M, Andreassen H, Eskildsen P, Langdahl B, Olgaard K: Bone mineral density and biochemical markers of bone turnover in patients with predialysis chronic renal failure. Kidney Int 56:1084-1093, 1999

42. Urena P, Hruby M, Ferreira A, Ang KS, De Vernejoul MC: Plasma total versus bone alkaline phosphatase as markers of bone turnover in hemodialysis patients. J Am Soc Nephrol 7:506-512, 1996

43. Couttenye MM, D'Haese PC, Van Hoof VO, Lemoniatou E, Goodman W, Verpooten GA, De Broe ME: Low serum levels of alkaline phosphatase of bone origin: a good marker of adynamic bone disease in haemodialysis patients. Nephrol Dial Transplant 11:1065-1072, 1996

44. Price PA, Parthemore JG, Deftos LJ: New biochemical marker for bone metabolism. Measurement by radioimmunoassay of bone GLA protein in the plasma of normal subjects and patients with bone disease. J Clin Invest 66:878-883, 1980

45. Ingram RT, Park YK, Clarke BL, Fitzpatrick LA: Age- and gender-related changes in the distribution of osteocalcin in the extracellular matrix of normal male and female bone. Possible involvement of osteocalcin in bone remodeling. J Clin Invest 93:989-997, 1994

46. Ducy P, Desbois C, Boyce B, Pinero G, Story B, Dunstan C, Smith E, Bonadio J, Goldstein S, Gundberg C, Bradley A, Karsenty G: Increased bone formation in osteocalcin-deficient mice. Nature 382:448-452, 1996

*47. Urena P, De Vernejoul MC: Circulating biochemical markers of bone remodeling in uremic patients. Kidney Int 55:2141-2156, 1999

48. Urena P, Ferreira A, Kung VT, Morieux C, Simon P, Ang KS, Souberbielle JC, Segre GV, Drueke TB, De Vernejoul MC: Serum pyridinoline as a specific marker of collagen breakdown and bone metabolism in hemodialysis patients. J Bone Miner Res 10:932-939, 1995

49. Charhon SA, Delmas PD, Malaval L, Chavassieux PM, Arlot M, Chapuy MC, Meunier PJ: Serum bone Gla-protein in renal osteodystrophy: comparison with bone histomorphometry. J Clin Endocrinol Metab 63:892-897, 1986

50. Morishita T, Nomura M, Hanaoka M, Saruta T, Matsuo T, Tsukamoto Y: A new assay method that detects only intact osteocalcin. Two-step non-invasive diagnosis to predict adynamic bone disease in haemodialysed patients. Nephrol Dial Transplant 15:659-667, 2000

51. Coen G, Mazzaferro S, Ballanti P, Bonucci E, Bondatti F, Manni M, Pasquali M, Perruzza I, Sardella D, Spurio A: Procollagen type I C-terminal extension peptide in predialysis chronic renal failure. Am J Nephrol 12:246-251, 1992

52. Hamdy NA, Risteli J, Risteli L, Harris S, Beneton MN, Brown CB, Kanis JA: Serum type I procollagen peptide: a non-invasive index of bone formation in patients on haemodialysis? Nephrol Dial Transplant 9:511-516, 1994

53. Ibrahim S, Mojiminiyi S, Barron JL: Pyridinium crosslinks in patients on haemodialysis and continuous ambulatory peritoneal dialysis. Nephrol Dial Transplant 10:2290-2294, 1995

54. Mazzaferro S, Pasquali M, Ballanti P, Bonucci E, Costantini S, Chicca S, De Meo S, Perruzza I, Sardella D, Taggi F, .: Diagnostic value of serum peptides of collagen synthesis and degradation in dialysis renal osteodystrophy. Nephrol Dial Transplant 10:52-58, 1995

55. Igarashi Y, Lee MY, Matsuzaki S: Acid phosphatases as markers of bone metabolism. J Chromatogr B Analyt Technol Biomed Life Sci 781:345-358, 2002

56. Nowak Z, Konieczna M, Wankowicz Z: [Tartrate-resistant acid phosphatase—TRAP 5b—as a modern bone resorption marker in patients with irreversible renal failure treated with dialysis]. Pol Merkuriusz Lek 17:138-141, 2004

57. Alfrey AC, Hegg A, Craswell P: Metabolism and toxicity of aluminum in renal failure. Am J Clin Nutr 33:1509-1516, 1980

58. D'Haese PC, Clement JP, Elseviers MM, Lamberts LV, Van de Vyver FL, Visser WJ, De Broe ME: Value of serum aluminium monitoring in dialysis patients: a multicentre study. Nephrol Dial Transplant 5:45-53, 1990

59. Milliner DS, Nebeker HG, Ott SM, Andress DL, Sherrard DJ, Alfrey AC, Slatopolsky EA, Coburn JW: Use of the deferoxamine infusion test in the diagnosis of aluminum-related osteodystrophy. Ann Intern Med 101:775-779, 1984

60. Smith AJ, Faugere MC, Abreo K, Fanti P, Julian B, Malluche HH: aluminum-related bone disease in mild and advanced renal failure: evidence for high prevalence and morbidity and studies on etiology and diagnosis. Am J Nephrol 6:275-283, 1986

61. Gejyo F, Yamada T, Odani S, Nakagawa Y, Arakawa M, Kunitomo T, Kataoka H, Suzuki M, Hirasawa Y, Shirahama T: A new form of amyloid protein associated with chronic hemodialysis was identified as beta 2-microglobulin. Biochem Biophys Res Commun 129:701-706, 1985

62. Koch KM: Dialysis-related amyloidosis. Kidney Int 41:1416-1429, 1992

63. Karlsson FA, Groth T, Sege K, Wibell L, Peterson PA: Turnover in humans of beta 2-microglobulin: the constant chain of HLA-antigens. Eur J Clin Invest 10:293-300, 1980

64. Kleinman KS, Coburn JW: Amyloid syndromes associated with hemodialysis. Kidney Int 35:567-575, 1989

65. Kay J: Review: Beta2-microglobulin amyloidosis. Int J Exp Clin Invest 4:187-211, 1997

*66. Sprague SM, Moe SM: Clinical manifestations and pathogenesis of dialysis-related amyloidosis. Semin Dial 9:360-369, 1996

67. Kuchle C, Fricke H, Held E, Schiffl H: High-flux hemodialysis postpones clinical manifestation of dialysis-related amyloidosis. Am J Nephrol 16:484-488, 1996

*68. Fukagawa M, Kitaoka M, Inazawa T, Kurokawa K: Imaging of the parathyroid in chronic renal failure: diagnostic and therapeutic aspects. Curr Opin Nephrol Hypertens 6:349-355, 1997

*69. Drueke TB: Cell biology of parathyroid gland hyperplasia in chronic renal failure. J Am Soc Nephrol 11:1141-1152, 2000

70. Fukuda N, Tanaka H, Tominaga Y, Fukagawa M, Kurokawa K, Seino Y: Decreased 1,25-dihydroxyvitamin D3 receptor density is associated with a more severe form of parathyroid hyperplasia in chronic uremic patients. J Clin Invest 92:1436-1443, 1993

71. Tominaga Y, Sato K, Tanaka Y, Numano M, Uchida K, Takagi H: Histopathology and pathophysiology of secondary hyperparathyroidism due to chronic renal failure. Clin Nephrol 44 Suppl 1:S42-S47, 1995

72. Fukagawa M, Kitaoka M, Yi H, Fukuda N, Matsumoto T, Ogata E, Kurokawa K: Serial evaluation of parathyroid size by ultrasonography is another useful marker for the long-term prognosis of calcitriol pulse therapy in chronic dialysis patients. Nephron 68:221-228, 1994

73. Fukagawa M, Tominaga Y, Kitaoka M, Kakuta T, Kurokawa K: Medical and surgical aspects of parathyroidectomy. Kidney Int Suppl 73:S65-S69, 1999

74. Tominaga Y: Surgical management of secondary hyperparathyroidism in uremia. Am J Med Sci 317:390-397, 1999

75. Tominaga Y, Tanaka Y, Sato K, Numano M, Uchida K, Falkmer U, Grimelius L, Johansson H, Takagi H: Recurrent renal hyperparathyroidism and DNA analysis of autografted parathyroid tissue. World J Surg 16:595-602, 1992

76. Fukagawa M, Kitaoka M, Kurokawa K: Ultrasonographic intervention of parathyroid hyperplasia in chronic dialysis patients: a theoretical approach. Nephrol Dial Transplant 11 Suppl 3:125-129, 1996

77. Kitaoka M: Ultrasonographic diagnosis of parathyroid glands and percutaneous ethanol injection therapy. Nephrol Dial Transplant 18 Suppl 3:ii27-ii30, 2003

78. Gotthardt M, Lohmann B, Behr TM, Bauhofer A, Franzius C, Schipper ML, Wagner M, Hoffken H, Sitter H, Rothmund M, Joseph K, Nies C: Clinical value of parathyroid scintigraphy with technetium-99m methoxyisobutylisonitrile: discrepancies in clinical data and a systematic metaanalysis of the literature. World J Surg 28:100-107, 2004

79. Olaizola I, Zingraff J, Heuguerot C, Fajardo L, Leger A, Lopez J, Acuna G, Petraglia A, Alvarez A, Caorsi H, Drueke T, Ambrosoni P: [(99m)Tc]-sestamibi parathyroid scintigraphy in chronic haemodialysis patients: static and dynamic explorations. Nephrol Dial Transplant 15:1201-1206, 2000

80. Weber ALUMINUM, Randolph G, Aksoy FG: The thyroid and parathyroid glands. CT and MR imaging and correlation with pathology and clinical findings. Radiol Clin North Am 38:1105-1129, 2000

*81. Llach F, Bover J: Renal Osteodystophies, in Brenner BM (ed): The Kidney, chap 51. 2000, pp 2103-2186

82. Black DM, Cummings SR, Genant HK, Nevitt MC, Palermo L, Browner W: Axial and appendicular bone density predict fractures in older women. J Bone Miner Res 7:633-638, 1992

83. Melton LJ, III, Atkinson EJ, O'Fallon WM, Wahner HW, Riggs BL: Long-term fracture prediction by bone mineral assessed at different skeletal sites. J Bone Miner Res 8:1227-1233, 1993

84. Stein MS, Packham DK, Ebeling PR, Wark JD, Becker GJ: Prevalence and risk factors for osteopenia in dialysis patients. Am J Kidney Dis 28:515-522, 1996

85. Alem AM, Sherrard DJ, Gillen DL, Weiss NS, Beresford SA, Heckbert SR, Wong C, Stehman-Breen C: Increased risk of hip fracture among patients with end-stage renal disease. Kidney Int 58:396-399, 2000

*86. Coco M, Rush H: Increased incidence of hip fractures in dialysis patients with low serum parathyroid hormone. Am J Kidney Dis 36:1115-1121, 2000

87. Atsumi K, Kushida K, Yamazaki K, Shimizu S, Ohmura A, Inoue T: Risk factors for vertebral fractures in renal osteodystrophy. Am J Kidney Dis 33:287-293, 1999

88. Fontaine MA, Albert A, Dubois B, Saint-Remy A, Rorive G: Fracture and bone mineral density in hemodialysis patients. Clin Nephrol 54:218-226, 2000

89. Jamal SA, Chase C, Goh YI, Richardson R, Hawker GA: Bone density and heel ultrasound testing do not identify patients with dialysis-dependent renal failure who have had fractures. Am J Kidney Dis 39:843-849, 2002

90. Yamaguchi T, Kanno E, Tsubota J, Shiomi T, Nakai M, Hattori S: Retrospective study on the usefulness of radius and lumbar bone density in the separation of hemodialysis patients with fractures from those without fractures. Bone 19:549-555, 1996

91. Piraino B, Chen T, Cooperstein L, Segre G, Puschett J: Fractures and vertebral bone mineral density in patients with renal osteodystrophy. Clin Nephrol 30:57-62, 1988

*92. Schober HC, Han ZH, Foldes AJ, Shih MS, Rao DS, Balena R, Parfitt AM: Mineralized bone loss at different sites in dialysis patients: implications for prevention. J Am Soc Nephrol 9:1225-1233, 1998

*Suggested Reading

MORBIDITY AND MORTALITY

Geoffrey A. Block

John Cunningham

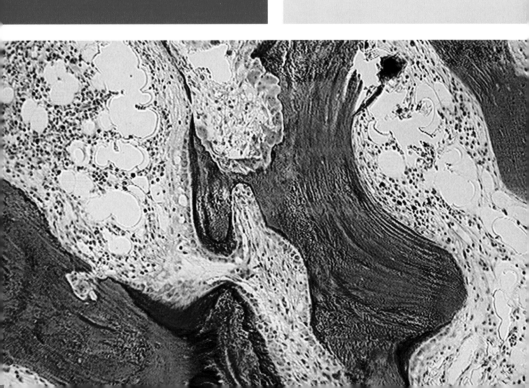

CHAPTER 4

MORBIDITY AND MORTALITY ASSOCIATED WITH DISORDERS OF BONE AND MINERAL METABOLISM IN CKD

Geoffrey A. Block and John Cunningham

Despite remarkable advances in the technical ability to provide dialysis, the all-cause mortality rate for patients on dialysis has, since 1985, decreased by a modest 9%-12%.[1] In fact, when adjusted for vintage, all-cause mortality has not improved between 1994 and 2002, and the adjusted mortality rate of patients on dialysis remains in excess of 240/1,000 patient-years.[1] To put this in perspective, a 60-year-old patient on hemodialysis has a life expectancy of 4.3 years as compared to a life expectancy of 22 years for a peer with normal kidney function. For younger patients, the increase in relative risk (RR) is much greater—life expectancy for a 25- to 29-year-old falls from an average of 51 years to 13 years in patients requiring kidney replacement therapy. Nearly 50% of dialysis patients are reported to die from cardiovascular (CV) events and, over the last decade, there has been a 7% *increase* in admission rates for patients with CV disease.[1]

While there is widespread recognition of the scope of the CV disease problem in patients with chronic kidney disease (CKD), its etiology and pathogenesis remain unclear. Unarguably, the burden of traditional CV risk factors is quite high in this population and the presence of CV morbidity at the time of initiation of dialysis is increasing. However, the classical risk factors for atherosclerotic vascular disease do not explain the 10- to 100-fold increase in CV event rate in patients requiring dialysis, and the search for pertinent and modifiable CV risk factors continues. This chapter will describe the expanding body of literature associating abnormalities in bone and mineral metabolism with CV morbidity and mortality in the dialysis population.

A consistent barrier to a deeper understanding of the potential role of disorders of bone and mineral metabolism, as an explanation for the increased CV risk, is the fact that essentially all of the data describing these associations come from cross-sectional, retrospective, or historical, prospective observational trials. Although some of these associations have biologically plausible mechanisms supporting their validity, there are no prospective randomized or interventional clinical trials that confirm that active intervention to modify plasma levels of calcium, phosphorus, or parathyroid hormone (PTH) levels will improve mortality. Despite extensive statistical adjustments and various statistical modeling techniques, all of these observational data are susceptible to errors as a result of missing potential confounders and confounding by indication. The results of prospective, randomized clinical trials using hormone replacement therapy in postmenopausal women, which conflicted with numerous analyses of epidemiological observational data, highlight the dangers of assigning a causal relationship to even statistically strong observations.

Nonetheless, almost all international clinical practice guidelines are largely based on observations that show a direct relationship between abnormal plasma calcium, phosphorus, and PTH, and morbidity and mortality in patients with kidney failure. This chapter will address data describing hard clinical endpoints such as hospitalization and mortality, as well as the intermediate (surrogate) endpoint of vascular calcification. It is now well established that the presence and extent of vascular calcification is associated with CV events and with all-cause mortality in patients on hemodialysis.[2] (*Refer to Chapter 5 for a more thorough discussion of vascular calcification and its relationship to outcomes, such as arterial stiffness/pulse wave velocity, CV events, and mortality.*)

PHOSPHORUS

Plasma phosphorus has been identified as a risk factor for vascular calcification, valvular calcification, all-cause and CV hospitalization, and all-cause and CV mortality. The potential effect of phosphorus on mortality in dialysis patients was originally identified in 1990 when it was shown that both low and high phosphorus were associated with mortality in univariate analysis.[3] In 1998, investigators at the United States Renal Data System (USRDS) reported a 6% increase in mortality per 1 mg/dL (0.32 mmol/L) increase in plasma phosphorus as a continuous variable.[4] Similar risk estimates were confirmed by three other groups. An 8% increase in the RR of death at 1 year per 1 mg/dL (0.32 mmol/L) increase in plasma phosphorus was described in a cohort of 37,000 patients on hemodialysis (p<0.001).[5] Data from the Dialysis Outcomes and Practice Patterns Study (DOPPS)—a large, international sample of dialysis patients—show a 4 % increase in mortality per 1 mg/dL (0.32 mmol/L) increase in plasma phosphorus (p<0.0001).[6] Most recently, Canadian investigators found that—after adjustment for demographic variables, dialysis type and adequacy, hemoglobin and albumin—plasma phosphorus independently predicted mortality with a RR of 1.56 per 1 mmol/L (p=.004).[7] Thus, numerous independent investigators have described a direct association between plasma phosphorus and survival as a continuous variable. The threshold of plasma phosphorus at which mortality is increased was recently described in a cohort of nearly 40,000 prevalent hemodialysis patients. When plasma phosphorus rose above 5 mg/dL (1.6 mmol/L), a significant increase in RR of death was observed, suggesting that normal phosphorus levels were associated with the most favorable outcome.[8] Consistent with this result, it was recently reported that elevations in plasma phosphorus >3.5 mg/dL (1.12 mmol/L) in patients with CKD not yet on dialysis were independently associated with mortality, and that each 1.0 mg/dL (0.32 mmol/L) increment in plasma phosphorus was linearly associated with increased mortality risk (p<0.001).[9]

Several groups have suggested that elevations in plasma phosphorus are associated specifically with CV mortality. In an analysis of data from the USRDS, a 20% increase in the risk of sudden death associated with plasma phosphorus >6.5 mg/dL (2.08 mmol/L), and a 41% increase in death from coronary artery disease were reported.[10] More recently, data from DOPPS found a 10% increase in CV death per 1 mg/dL (0.32 mmol/L) increase in plasma phosphorus, after extensive statistical adjustment.[6] As would be expected, it appears that patients with previous evidence of CV disease are at a greatly exaggerated risk of CV death associated with elevations in plasma phosphorus, particularly when it is also associated with elevations in plasma calcium (Figure 1).

FIGURE 1. RELATIVE CORONARY MORTALITY RISK BY CALCIUM AND PHOSPHORUS

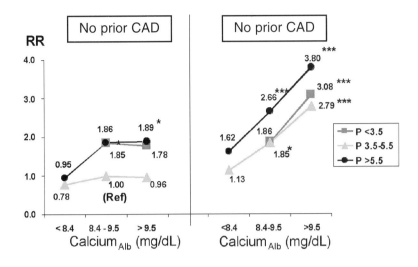

* p=0.01-0.05, *** p<0.001; Adjusted for factors shown above plus age, sex, black race, cause of CKD, years on dialysis, smoking (active), UFR, BMI, spKt/V, Hgb, albumin, iPTH, cholesterol, triglycerides, % lymphocytes and neutrophils, vascular access, and 14 summary comorbid conditions. Calcuim-ALB = albumin-corrected calcium. Reprinted with permission of Dr. Fritz Port.

Although there have been no prospective trials demonstrating that reductions in plasma phosphorus are associated with improvements in survival, observational data confirm that control of plasma phosphorus is a modifiable risk factor associated with long-term survival of dialysis patients.[11] In a recent retrospective, observational study in a cohort of incident hemodialysis patients, it was reported that administration of activated vitamin D attenuated the relationship between plasma phosphorus and mortality.[12] However, it has been suggested that dialysis duration and the complex interaction between PTH, calcium, and phosphorus accounts for at least part of this paradoxical finding. Investigators noted that incident patients with low PTH had the most unfavorable outcome and thus would have been less likely to have received vitamin D.[7]

The observations regarding a direct relationship between plasma phosphorus and mortality are supported by evidence showing that increases in plasma phosphorus are associated with morbid events (e.g., vascular calcification and hospitalization). In a cross-sectional analysis of maintenance hemodialysis patients, the extent of coronary artery calcification was reported to be directly associated with higher plasma phosphorus concentration (p=0.005), with each 1 mg/dL (0.32 mmol/L) increase in plasma phosphorus conferring a risk for calcification equivalent to 2.5 years of dialysis therapy.[13] Plasma phosphorus was also directly associated with aortic calcification (p=0.007). In an analysis of young hemodialysis patients, plasma phosphorus concentration was higher in subjects with coronary calcification, and was positively correlated with changes in coronary calcium scores using serial electron beam computed tomography.[14] Similar findings were reported in an analysis of risk factors associated with the extent of vascular calcification in which there was a significant relationship between plasma phosphorus levels and the number of calcified arteries (p<0.01).[15] As mentioned previously, the extent of vascular calcification is a strong independent predictor of mortality in patients on hemodialysis.[2] It is clear, however, that plasma phosphorus levels alone are not sufficient to predict progressive vascular calcification. Despite equivalent phosphorus control, subjects receiving calcium-containing phosphate binders were more likely to experience progressive coronary and aortic calcification compared to those receiving sevelamer hydrocholoride.[16]

Recent observational data from a large dialysis provider (n=40,538) in the United States have provided a direct relationship between increases in plasma phosphorus and both all-cause and CV hospitalization as shown in Figure 2.[8]

FIGURE 2. RELATIVE RISK OF ALL CAUSE AND CARDIOVASCULAR HOSPITALIZATIONS BY SERUM PHOSPHORUS

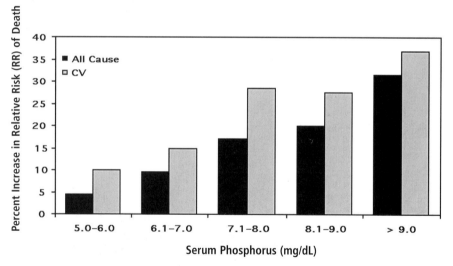

Multivariable analysis adjusted for age, gender, race or ethnicity, diabetes, vintage, body weight, URR, serum albumin, creatinine, predialysis BUN, bicarbonate, cholesterol, hemoglobin, ferritin, and aluminum. *Adapted from: Block GA, Klassen PS, Lazarus JM, Ofsthun N, Lowrie E, Chertow GM: Mineral metabolism, mortality, and morbidity in maintenance hemodialysis. J Am Soc Nephrol 15:2208-2218, 2004.*

CALCIUM

Until recently, there was no evidence of an independent effect of plasma calcium on mortality or CV events in patients requiring hemodialysis. In fact, at least one group reported that patients with plasma calcium <8.8 mg/dL (2.2 mmol/L) had an *increased* mortality rate, while data from the USRDS failed to find any statistically significant increase in mortality associated with increases in plasma calcium.[4;17] Each of these reports was compromised by the small numbers of patients and limited ability to adjust for important covariates. More recently, investigators reported a 16% increase in 1-year mortality associated with a 1 mg/dL (0.25 mmol/L) increase in plasma calcium in a cohort of 37,000 hemodialysis patients; in a similar database of nearly 40,000 hemodialysis patients, a direct relationship between plasma calcium level and mortality has been described.[5;8] In the fully adjusted model, each 1 mg/dL (0.25 mmol/L) increase in plasma calcium (derived from an average of values obtained over a 3-month period of time) was associated with approximately a 20% increase in mortality. A striking—and in some respects, counterintuitive—observation is that this effect was not confined to the high physiological and supraphysiological range but extended right across (and even slightly below) the "normal" range (Figure 3). It was independent of plasma phosphorus and PTH and, in fact, the RR associated with increases in plasma calcium was consistent even in cohorts of subjects with normal plasma phosphorus levels. Data from DOPPS confirm a strong association between albumin-corrected plasma calcium and both all-cause and CV mortality (Figure 4).[6]

FIGURE 3. RELATIVE RISK OF MORTALITY BY SERUM CALCIUM

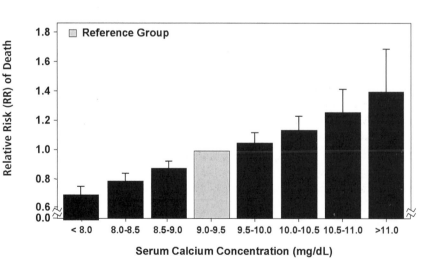

Multivariable analysis adjusted for age, gender, race or ethnicity, diabetes, vintage, body weight, URR, serum albumin, creatinine, predialysis BUN, bicarbonate, cholesterol, hemoglobin, ferritin, and aluminum. *Adapted from: Block GA, Klassen PS, Lazarus JM, Ofsthun N, Lowrie E, Chertow GM: Mineral metabolism, mortality, and morbidity in maintenance hemodialysis. J Am Soc Nephrol 15:2208-2218, 2004.*

FIGURE 4. RELATIVE RISK OF MORTALITY BY CORRECTED CALCIUM

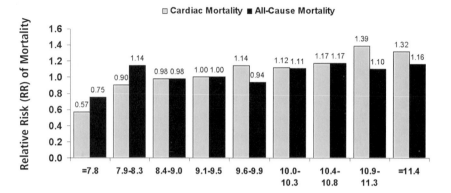

Albumin-corrected calcium (mg/dL)

DOPPS I data (1996-2000). Model stratified by country, corrected for facility clustering, and adjusted for age, race, gender, years with ESRD, BMI, 14 summary comorbid conditions, dialysate calcium, serum iPTH, phosphorus, albumin, vitamin D use, phosphate binder use, and prior parathyroidectomy. n= 12,114. Reprinted with permission from: Young EW, Akiba T, Albert J, McCarthy J, Kerr PG, Mendelssohn DC, Jadoul M: Magnitude and Impact of Abnormal Mineral Metabolism in Hemodialysis Patients in the Dialysis Outcomes and Practice Patterns Study (DOPPS). Am J Kidney Dis 44:S34-S38, 2004

As shown earlier in Figure 1, the increase in risk associated with increases in plasma calcium is particularly evident in subjects with underlying coronary artery disease. Again, it is evident that the RR associated with increasing plasma calcium is demonstrable even within the normal range and certainly when calcium levels rise above the K/DOQI threshold of 9.5 mg/dL (2.38 mmol/L). As described previously for phosphorus, it has been suggested that the relative mortality risk associated with increases in plasma calcium is attenuated in incident dialysis patients given activated vitamin D.[12] When examined in the DOPPS database of prevalent patients, investigators could find no such survival benefit associated with the use of activated vitamin D, and currently this hypothesis remains unproven.[6;18]

Increases in plasma calcium have been implicated in the molecular mechanism underlying vascular calcification.[19] There is some corroborating evidence in the dialysis population for such a relationship; however, many authors report that average plasma calcium values are a poor marker for the presence of vascular calcification and do not reliably discriminate between patients undergoing progressive calcification and those who remain noncalcified. In a study of young dialysis patients, no difference in mean plasma calcium was found in patients with or without coronary calcification.[14] Similarly, investigators were unable to show any relationship between plasma calcium and the number of calcified arterial sites.[15] In a randomized trial comparing the rate of progressive vascular calcification in prevalent hemodialysis patients, those with a mean time-averaged plasma calcium >9.5 mg/dL (2.38 mmol/L) who were randomized to calcium-containing phosphate binders experienced progressive increases in both coronary and aortic calcification. Those who were given calcium-containing phosphate binders but maintained a time-averaged calcium <9.5 mg/dL (2.38 mmol/L) did not.[20] The baseline data from this same trial found a strong association between baseline plasma calcium and coronary artery but not aortic calcification score, with each 1 mg/dL (0.25 mmol/L) increase in plasma calcium conferring a risk for calcification equivalent to 5 years of dialysis therapy.[21]

Plasma calcium levels do not necessarily reflect actual calcium balance, and it is likely that many patients on hemodialysis are in long-term positive calcium balance due to the use of calcium-containing phosphate binders, activated vitamin D, and a moderate to high dialysate calcium bath. Any such relationship that may exist between calcium intake (via the gastrointestinal tract or dialysate) and prevailing plasma calcium concentration is likely to be perturbed by calcimimetic therapy which, by lowering plasma calcium concentration, may lead to a false sense of security. Several investigators have reported that prescribed dose of calcium (an indirect estimate of calcium load) is an independent risk factor for progressive vascular calcification.[14-16;20;22] Data from DOPPS suggest that, independent of plasma calcium, increased dialysate calcium concentration is associated with increased all-cause mortality [RR 1.13 per 1 mEq/L (0.5 mmol/L) increase, p=.01].[6;18] It has been suggested that the risk associated with calcium intake is a result of the inability of the skeleton to accommodate the augmented calcium load, thereby resulting in transient elevations in plasma calcium. This is particularly true in the setting of reduced bone remodeling, a clinical situation often associated with excessively reduced PTH. Supporting this proposed mechanism, it has been reported that patients with a biochemical profile of low PTH, high calcium, and high phosphorus have the highest mortality rate.[7] In a study of 58 patients undergoing iliac crest bone biopsy, patients with the lowest bone turnover were found to have the greatest evidence of systemic vascular calcification.[15]

CALCIUM-PHOSPHORUS PRODUCT

As one would expect from the discussion of phosphorus and calcium as isolated variables, there have been many reported associations of calcium-phosphorus product (CaxP) with progressive vascular calcification, valvular calcification, and mortality. It is unclear whether there is an *independent* risk associated with elevations in CaxP after consideration of the individual laboratory abnormalities. It has been suggested that the circulating level of inhibitors of calcification may modify the likelihood of producing an elevated CaxP, and that "normal" CaxP levels may be the result of rapid tissue calcification.[23] Certainly the introduction into clinical practice of calcimimetics, which directly reduce plasma calcium concentration, will facilitate the simultaneous occurrence of a CaxP within "desirable" range, while each unique variable

FIGURE 5. RELATIVE RISK OF MORTALITY BY CALCIUM X PHOSPHORUS PRODUCT

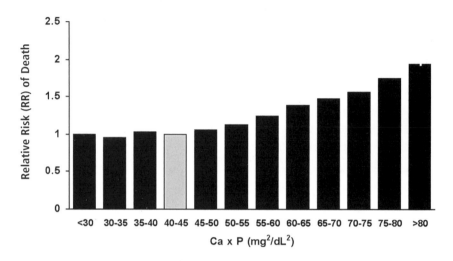

*Multivariable analysis adjusted for age, gender, race or ethnicity, diabetes, vintage, body weight, URR, serum albumin, creatinine, predialysis BUN, bicarbonate, cholesterol, hemoglobin, ferritin, and aluminum. *Adapted from: Block GA, Klassen PS, Lazarus JM, Ofsthun N, Lowrie E, Chertow GM: Mineral metabolism, mortality, and morbidity in maintenance hemodialysis. J Am Soc Nephrol 15:2208-2218, 2004.*

may, in fact, be abnormal (low calcium and high phosphorus). Recent observational data suggest that a CaxP >45 mg^2/dL^2 is associated with an increased RR of death (Figure 5).[8]

In an analysis of the DOPPS data set, investigators have reported a 3% increase in the RR of all-cause death per 5 mg^2/dL^2 increase in CaxP and a 6% increase in the RR of CV death.[6;18] Similar to data presented earlier with the individual variables of calcium and phosphorus, there appears to be a unique risk for CV death associated with elevations in CaxP in subjects with prior evidence of atherosclerotic vascular disease.

Parathyroid Hormone
The alterations in parathyroid gland function that occur in CKD have significant effects on bone histology and have additional systemic effects in multiple organ systems. These effects have been discussed in more detail in Chapter 3.

The relationship between plasma PTH levels and mortality is quite complex. Both low and high PTH are associated with elevations in plasma calcium and phosphorus, and have been associated with adverse outcomes. In general, epidemiological analyses find that—after adjustment for case mix and laboratory variables (including calcium and phosphorus)—only patients with severe hyperparathyroidism are at increased risk of mortality. Using a large U.S. dialysis chain database of 40,538 patients, there is a significant increase in mortality above a PTH level of 600 pg/mL, which is driven primarily by an 18% increase in mortality risk observed in patients with a PTH level >900 pg/mL (99 pmol/L).[8] PTH values >600 pg/mL were also associated with CV hospitalization, fracture, and all-cause hospitalization. Globally, data from DOPPS find a statistically significant 1% increase in the RR of all-cause mortality per 100 pg/mL (11 pmol/L) increase in PTH and a 2 % increase in CV mortality (p=.007) (Table 1).[18] Both of these analyses adjust for plasma calcium and phosphorus in order to isolate the independent effects of PTH. However, hypercalcemia and hyperphosphatemia are direct consequences of both elevated and suppressed PTH, and statistical adjustment may therefore confound the actual relationship between severity of secondary hyperparathyroidism (SHPT) and clinical outcome. In a more clinically relevant analysis of combinations of PTH, calcium, and phosphorus, the most unfavorable outcome (increased mortality) was seen in patients with a combination of low PTH, high calcium, and high phosphorus (Figure 6).[7]

TABLE 1. RELATIONSHIP BETWEEN MORTALITY AND LABORATORY PARAMETERS

Laboratory Measure	RR	95% CI	p-value
Phosphorus (per 1 mg/dL or 0.32 mmol/L)	1.04	1.02-1.06	<0.001
Albumin-Corrected Calcium (per 1 mg/dL or 0.25 mmol/L)	1.10	1.06-1.15	<0.001
Calcium-Phosphorus Product (per 1 mg²/dL²)	1.01	1.00-1.01	<0.001
iPTH (per 100 pg/mL or 11 pmol/L)	1.01	1.00-1.02	0.04
Dialysate Calcium (per 1 mEq/L or 0.5 mmol/L)	1.12	1.02-1.23	0.02

Models stratified by country and adjusted for age, sex, race, time on dialysis, hemoglobin, spKt/V, albumin, and 14 summary comorbid conditions, accounted for facility clustering (n=16,306). Abbreviations: RR, Relative Risk; CI, Confidence Interval. In: *Young EW, Albert JM, Satayathum S, Goodkin DA, Pisoni RL, Akiba T, Akizawa T, Kurokawa K, Bommer J, Piera L, Port FK: Predictors and consequences of altered mineral metabolism: the Dialysis Outcomes and Practice Patterns Study. Kidney Int 67:1179-1187, 2005.*

FIGURE 6. SURVIVAL AS A FUNCTION OF CALCIUM, Pi, AND iPTH COMBINATIONS

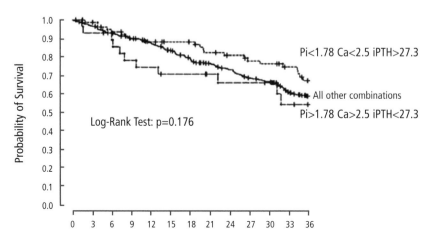

These authors show that the relative risks of various combinations of calcium, phosphorus, and PTH vary with dialysis duration. Their data suggest that incident patients are at particular risk with high phosphorus, high calcium, and low PTH, while patients who have survived greater than 18 months seem to have increased risk particularly associated with increased calcium. This important observation likely underlies the discrepant reports regarding the effect of PTH on survival.

CONCLUSIONS

It is clear that disturbances in bone and mineral metabolism are closely associated with adverse CV outcomes in patients requiring dialysis. Cause-and-effect relationships are harder to establish, but available evidence suggests that they are quite likely. The precise mechanisms underlying this linkage are unknown but are likely related, in some degree, to an effect on vascular calcification. Unfortunately, the ability to reach the recommended target ranges shown in Table 2 is poor.[6] In a point prevalence analysis, nearly 20% of the DOPPS population did not meet a single K/DOQI guideline for mineral metabolism and only 5% of patients were able to meet all four guidelines. Data from this observational trial show that only modest improvements have occurred over the last 5 years in achieving these biochemical targets. Globally, nearly 50% of patients continue to have a plasma phosphorus >5.5 mg/dL (1.76 pmol/L). Of great concern, practice-pattern analysis suggests that patients with overtly low PTH continue to receive therapy with vitamin D (thus placing them at risk for hypercalcemia and hyperphosphatemia), while a substantial proportion of subjects with overtly high PTH and otherwise acceptable calcium and phosphorus levels are not receiving any therapy for their SHPT.[18]

When evaluating the relative importance of mutable risk factors in hemodialysis patients, we have found that the attributable risk associated with disorders of mineral metabolism, defined as phosphorus >5.0 mg/dL (1.6 mmol/L), calcium >10 mg/dL (2.5 mmol/L), and PTH >600 pg/mL (66 pmol/L) are higher than those associated with inefficient dialysis (urea reduction ratio <65%), or anemia (hemoglobin <11 g/dL or 6.83 mmol/L). Given the current evidence of the relative adverse effects of phosphorus, calcium, and PTH, treatment strategies that concentrate solely on PTH without adequate consideration for the effect on calcium and phosphorus seem ill-advised. A post-hoc analysis of patients with SHPT treated with cinacalcet in addition to their usual regimen showed significant improvements in plasma calcium, phosphorus, and PTH, and additionally found a favorable effect on clinically relevant endpoints including fracture, parathyroidectomy, CV hospitalization, and quality of life.[24] Intervention studies, however, are certainly needed to define the best treatment strategies. Until the results of these studies are available, it is reasonable to assume that the most favorable outcomes are likely to be realized in those patients in whom calcium intake is modest and plasma calcium and phosphorus are normalized.

TABLE 2. ACHIEVING NKF K/DOQI TARGET RANGES FOR MINERAL METABOLISM

Measurement (n1/n2)	Range[1]	Patients (%)		p-value
		1999	2002	
	0	19.6	17.8	
Number of lab values within guideline ranges (1443/1697)	At least 1	80.4	82.2	0.08
	At least 2	54.8	57.6	
	At least 3	25.3	27.5	
	All 4	5.4	5.5	

Point-prevalent cross-section for DOPPS I and II; n1/n2 = DOPPS I/DOPPS II sample size; [1] NKF K/DOQI guideline target range. In: *Young EW, Akiba T, Albert J, McCarthy J, Kerr PG, Mendelsohn DC, Jadoul M: Magnitude and Impact of Abnormal Mineral Metabolism in Hemodialysis Patients in the Dialysis Outcomes and Practice Patterns Study (DOPPS). Am J Kidney Dis 44:S34-S38, 2004.*

REFERENCES

1. USRDS 2004 annual data report. Am J Kidney Dis 45:8-280, 2005

2. Blacher J, Guerin AP, Pannier B, Marchais SJ, London AM: Arterial Calcifications, Arterial Stiffness, and Cardiovascular Risk in End Stage Renal Disease. Hypertension 38:938-942, 2001

3. Lowrie EG, Lew NJ: Death risk in hemodialysis patients: the predictive value of commonly measured variables and an evaluation of death rate differences between facilities. Am J Kidney Dis 15:458-482, 1990

4. Block GA, Hulbert-Shearon TE, Levin NW, Port FK: Association of serum phosphorus and calcium x phosphate product with mortality risk in chronic hemodialysis patients: a national study. Am J Kidney Dis 31:607-617, 1998

5. Klassen PS, Lowrie EG, Reddan DN, DeLong ER, Coladonato JA, Szezech LA, Lazarus JM, Owen WF: Association Between Pulse Pressure and Mortality in Patients Undergoing Maintenance Hemodialysis. JAMA 287:1548-1555, 2002

*6. Young EW, Akiba T, Albert J, McCarthy J, Kerr PG, Mendelssohn DC, Jadoul M: Magnitude and Impact of Abnormal Mineral Metabolism in Hemodialysis Patients in the Dialysis Outcomes and Practice Patterns Study (DOPPS). Am J Kidney Dis 44:S34-S38, 2004

*7. Stevens LA, Djurdjev O, Cardew S, Cameron EC, Levin A: Calcium, Phosphate, and Parathyroid Hormone Levels in Combination and as a function of dialysis duration predict mortality: evidence for the complexity of the association between mineral metabolism and outcomes. J Am Soc Nephrol 15:770-779, 2004

*8. Block GA, Klassen PS, Lazarus JM, Ofsthun N, Lowrie E, Chertow GM: Mineral metabolism, mortality, and morbidity in maintenance hemodialysis. J Am Soc Nephrol 15:2208-2218, 2004

9. Kestenbaum B, Sampson JN, Rudser KD, Patterson DJ, Seliger SL, Young B, Sherrard DJ, Andress DL: Serum phosphate levels and mortality risk among people with chronic kidney disease. J Am Soc Nephrol 16:520-528, 2005

10. Ganesh SK, Stack AG, Levin NW, Hulbert-Shearon TE, Port FK: Association of elevated serum PO4, CaxPO4 product, and parathyroid hormone with cardiac mortality risk in chronic hemodialysis patients. J Am Soc Nephrol 12:2131-2138, 2001

11. Okechukwu CN, Lopes AA, Stack AG, Feng S, Wolfe RA, Port FK: Impact of Years of Dialysis Therapy on Mortality Risk and the Characteristics of Longer Term Dialysis Survivors. Am J Kidney Dis 39:533-538, 2002

12. Teng M, Wolf M, Ofsthun N, Lazarus JM, Hernan MA, Camargo CA, Thadhani R: Activated injectable vitamin D and hemodialysis survival: a historical cohort study. J Am Soc Nephrol 16:1115-1125, 2005

13. Raggi P, Boulay A, Chasan-Tabar S, Amin NS, Dillon MA, Burke SK, Chertow GM: Cardiac Calcification in Adult Hemodialysis Patients. J Am Coll Cardiol 39:695-701, 2002

14. Goodman WG, Goldin J, Kuizon BD, Yoon C, Gales B, Sider D, Wang Y, Chung J, Emerick A, Greaser L, Elashoff RM, Salusky IB: Coronary artery calcification in young adults with end stage renal disease who are undergoing dialysis. N Engl J Med 342:1478-1483, 2000

*15. London GM, Marty C, Marchais SJ, Guerin AP, Metivier F, Vernejoul M-C: Arterial calcifications and bone histomorphometry in end stage renal disease. J Am Soc Nephrol 15:1943-1951, 2004

*16. Chertow GM, Burke SK, Raggi P: Sevelamer attenuates the progression of coronary and aortic calcification in hemodialysis patients. Kidney Int 62:245-252, 2002

17. Foley RN, Parfey PS, Harnett JD, Kent GM, Hu L, O'Dea R, Murray DC, Barre PE: Hypocalcemia, Morbidity and Mortality in End Stage Renal Disease. Am J Nephrol 16:386-393, 1996

18. Young EW, Albert JM, Satayathum S, Goodkin DA, Pisoni RL, Akiba T, Akizawa T, Kurokawa K, Bommer J, Piera L, Port FK: Predictors and consequences of altered mineral metabolism: the Dialysis Outcomes and Practice Patterns Study. Kidney Int 67:1179-1187, 2005

19. Yang H, Curinga G, Giachelli CM: Elevated extracellular calcium levels induce smooth muscle cell matrix mineralization in vitro. Kidney Int 66:1-7, 2004

20. Chertow GM, Raggi P, Chasan-Tabar S, Bommer J, Holzer H, Burke SK: Determinants of progressive vascular calcification in hemodialysis patients. Nephrol Dial Transplant 19:1489-1496, 2004

21. Raggi P, Rienmuller R, Chertow GM, Bommer J, Amin NS, Dillon MA, Burke SK: Cardiac calcification is prevalent and severe in ESRD patients as measured by electron beam CT scanning. J Am Soc Nephrol 2001 (Abstract)

22. Guerin AP, London GM, Marchais SJ, Metivier F: Arterial stiffening and vascular calcifications in end stage renal disease. Nephrol Dial Transplant1014-1021, 2000

23. Ketteler M, Brandenburg V, Jahnen-Dechent W, Westenfeld R, Floege J: Do not be misguided by guidelines: the calcium x phosphate product can be a Trojan horse. Nephrol Dial Transplant 20:673-677, 2005

24. Cunningham, J., Danese, M., Olson, K., Klassen, P., and Chertow, G. Effects of the calcimimetic cinacalcet HCl on cardiovascular disease, fracture and health related quality of life in secondary hyperparathyroidism. Kidney Int. 68 (4): 1793-1800, 2005

*Suggested Reading

VASCULAR CALCIFICATION IN CKD

Gerard M. London

Paolo Raggi

Keith A. Hruska

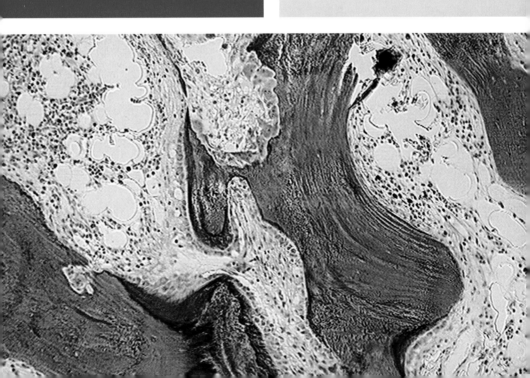

CHAPTER 5

VASCULAR CALCIFICATION IN CKD

Gerard M. London, Paolo Raggi and Keith A. Hruska

The incidence of cardiovascular (CV) mortality is markedly higher in Stage 5 CKD patients than in the general population as detailed in Chapter 4, and the relative prevalence of traditional risk factors does not fully explain this high rate of CV disease. Therefore, other factors specific to CKD must contribute to the high incidence of CV mortality.[1,2] Vascular calcification (VC) could be one of these factors. Studies have demonstrated that 60%-80% of prevalent dialysis patients have VC by some imaging methodology.[3-6] VC is an important component of CV disease in metabolic disorders, such as CKD and diabetes. The abnormalities in mineral metabolism in CKD and/or therapeutic measures used to manage them have been shown to contribute to the development of VC and to the high rates of CV morbidity and mortality.[4;7;8]

VC has historically been considered an unregulated, passive process that is part of the natural sequelae of atherosclerosis. However, recent studies have shown that VC is a complex, actively regulated process that resembles osteogenesis in bone.[9] This chapter discusses the mechanisms and clinical significance of VC in CKD. While this chapter will focus on VC, it should be noted that extraskeletal calcification can also affect other organs and soft tissues, such as the myocardium, skin, breasts, kidneys, and joints.

PATHOLOGY OF VASCULAR CALCIFICATION

VC can occur in the intima and the medial layer of arteries. While the processes leading to the development of the vascular disease clearly differs in these two arterial segments, there are insufficient data to determine if the mechanism is similar, due to lack of animal models.

Atherosclerotic Lesions

Calcification of the intimal layer occurs when minerals are deposited within or adjacent to atherosclerotic plaques in the intima of the vessel wall. Although it had been previously felt that calcification was a late process, occurring only in well-developed plaques, it is now known to occur earlier in the course of atherogenic disease. Intravascular ultrasound has demonstrated circumferential calcification that precedes luminal narrowing from protruding plaques. Calcified intimal atherosclerotic lesions are a progressive feature of atherosclerosis found in the general population, especially with aging. Atherogenic VC is accelerated in diabetes, and recent studies suggest that CKD also accelerates the development of atherogenic VC.[10]

Medial Wall Calcification

The second form of VC is characterized by diffuse mineral deposits within the medial wall of the arteries (medial calcinosis). This may occur in the presence or absence of atherosclerosis. While medial wall calcification (sometimes referred to as Mönckeberg's sclerosis) is character- istic of aging, it is significantly more pronounced in metabolic disorders such as diabetes and CKD.[9] These lesions have typically been described to occur in peripheral distal arteries, although medial calcification also likely contributes to large artery (aorta) calcification and subsequent stiffening (often called arteriosclerosis).

Calcific Uremic Arteriolopathy

Another form of medial VC is calcific uremic arteriolopathy (CUA), also referred to as calciphy- laxis. This disease is a necrotizing skin condition caused by medial calcification of cutaneous and subcutaneous arterioles. The arterial calcification and vascular occlusion leads to tissue ischemia and, eventually, necrosis.[11] CUA occurs almost exclusively in the CKD population and carries a high mortality rate. CUA can present as distal lesions with ulceration of the skin of the lower extremities (Figure 1), gangrene of the fingers and toes, or as proximal lesions affecting the skin and adipose tissue of the abdominal wall, thighs, and/or buttocks.[11] Risk factors for CUA include female gender, obesity, and low plasma albumin levels.[12]

MECHANISMS OF VASCULAR CALCIFICATIONS

There are now abundant data indicating that atherogenic VC is an active process that is regu- lated by a variety of genes and proteins, including several that are also directly involved in bone and mineral metabolism.[9] Various bone regulatory proteins, such as osteopontin, osteonectin, bone morphogenetic protein (BMP), parathyroid hormone-related protein (PTHrP), and the receptor for parathyroid hormone (PTH) and PTHrP can be detected in ather- osclerotic plaques as well as in medial calcifications.[13;14] It has been demonstrated in animal knockout models that VC can be induced by selective deletion of various genes, such as matrix gla protein (MGP) and osteoprotegerin.[15;16] These cumulative data strongly refute the historical perspective of extraskeletal calcification being a result of only passive precipitation due to oversaturation of minerals in the blood.

VC appears to follow a developmental process very similar to bone formation that includes extracellular matrix formation, initiation of apatite accumulation (nucleation), elaboration of matrix, and production of regulatory proteins. It has been suggested that physiological or pathological cell death may be the primary initiating event in the formation of VC, as apoptot- ic bodies that are not effectively cleared may act as the site of apatite nucleation (Figure 2).[17] In addition, elevations in extracellular calcium and phosphorus can directly induce mineraliza- tion, and the effects of the two ions are additive.[18]

FIGURE 1. DISTAL CALCIFIC UREMIC ARTERIOLOPATHY (CUA)

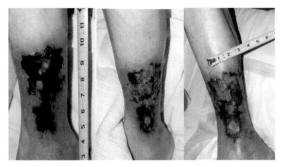

CUA usually begins as a hard, painful nodule under the skin, followed by central necrosis and eschar formation. The lesions progress rapidly as demonstrated in the 4 week progression of this large anterior tibial CUA lesion. (Adapted with permission from: R. Russell, M.A. Brookshire, M. Zekonis and S.M. Moe: Distal calcific uremic arteriolopathy in a hemodialysis patient responds to lowering of Ca P product and aggressive wound care. Vol. 58 - No. 3/2002, p. 240)

FIGURE 2. HYPOTHETICAL DEPICTION OF THE PATHOGENESIS OF VASCULAR CALCIFICATION

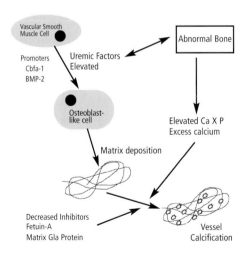

VSMCs are capable of dedifferentiating into osteoblast-like cells, a process that is stimulated by phosphorus and other uremic toxins. These osteoblast-like cells can produce bone matrix proteins resulting in tissue that resembles unmineralized osteoid. This osteoid-like tissue is capable of mineralizing, resulting in mineralized vasculature. The mineralizing process may be accelerated in the presence of elevated calcium-phosphorus product and/or increased calcium load. Reduction in endogenous inhibitors such as Fetuin A and Matrix Gla protein may also accelerate mineralization. Adapted from Reslerova and Moe.[17]

This calcification process involves differentiation of vascular smooth muscle cells (VSMC) into phenotypically distinct cells that have been shown to generate calcification *in vitro*.[9] VSMCs form nodules (similar to those produced by osteoblasts), synthesize bone-associated proteins, and form matrix vesicles. *In vitro*, the transformation of VSMCs into osteoblast-like cells (with subsequent mineralization) is induced or regulated by a variety of factors, including PTH, vitamin D, and calcium/phosphorus balance.[9] Other factors have been identified that may act as promoters or inhibitors of VC, including osteopontin, MGP, fetuin-A, BMP-2, and pyrophosphate (Table 1).[9;19] The severity of VC in CKD patients reflects the interplay between factors that either promote or inhibit calcium deposition in arterial tissue (Table 1).

TABLE 1. CELLULAR PROTEINS WITH POTENTIAL ROLES IN THE REGULATION OF VASCULAR CALCIFICATION

Inhibitors	Promoters	Nucleator
Matrix Gla protein	BMP-2	Collagen type I
Osteocalcin	Cbfa-1	
Osteopontin		
Osteoprotegerin		
PTHrP		
Fetuin A		
BMP-7		
Pyrophosphate		

Abbreviations: BMP, bone morphogenetic protein; PTHrP, parathyroid hormone-related protein.

Calcification Promoters and Inhibitors

The effect of phosphorus on VSMCs is particularly interesting in light of the increased morbidity and mortality associated with hyperphosphatemia in dialysis patients as detailed in Chapter 4.[7] Phosphorus was found to induce a concentration-dependent increase in VSMC calcification in vitro.[20] The phosphorus-stimulated apatite production can be completely inhibited by addition of agents that antagonize the cellular sodium-phosphate cotransport system.[20;21] Phosphorus may induce calcification by enhancing the expression of core-binding factor 1 (Cbfa1; also called Runx2), an osteoblast factor that stimulates differentiation of mesenchymal cells into osteoblasts.[13;20;21] Increased intracellular phosphate levels induce other osteoblast-like changes to VSMCs that are Cbfa-1 stimulated and implicated in the calcification process. These include increased expression of alkaline phosphatase, osteocalcin, and osteopontin, and the laying down of a collagen-rich extracellular matrix.[21;22]

Certain genes and proteins appear to serve as physiological inhibitors of soft-tissue calcification and VC (Table 1). Matrix Gla protein (MGP) is a local inhibitor that is expressed in VSMCs. The action of MGP is based on observations in knockout mice. Mice depleted of MGP develop dramatic calcification throughout the arterial tree, predominantly in the medial wall of arteries, and they die several months after birth due to arterial rupture and hemorrhage.[16] Thus, MGP appears to serve a fundamental physiological role as an inhibitor of VC. MGP may limit VC by binding to BMP-2, a promineralization factor.[23]

In dialysis patients, warfarin therapy has been identified as a risk factor for the development of uremic calcification.[12] It has been proposed that warfarin may led to a procalcifying environment by impeding normal metabolism and production of MGP.[24] Warfarin may affect the availability of vitamin K, which is a necessary coenzyme in the γ-carboxylation of MGP. In rats treated with warfarin, pathological changes consistent with tissue-specific impairments in MGP expression were noted, including calcification of epiphyseal growth plate cartilage and cardiac valves.[25] Based upon these observations, it is plausible that long-term warfarin therapy lowers the threshold for VC by reducing the synthesis of MGP in those already predisposed to this complication of chronic renal failure.

Fetuin-A (AHSG or α2-HS Glycoprotein) is a potential circulating VC inhibitor that is abundant in plasma. *In vitro*, Fetuin-A inhibits the formation and precipitation of calcium-phosphorus complexes, thus blocking the development of hydroxyapatite.[26] Mice deficient in Fetuin-A exhibited increased ectopic calcification.[27] Low levels of fetuin-A were associated with increased mortality,[28] increased carotid intimal-medial thickening,[29] and valvular calcification.[30] Fetuin-A is a reverse acute phase reactant, and low plasma Fetuin-A levels were associated with increased levels of the inflammatory marker CRP.[28]

In contrast to atherogenic calcification, medial calcification can occur in otherwise normal appearing arteries, and without inflammation. Expression of Cbfa-1, the osteoblast-specific transcription factor, has been demonstrated in human blood vessels from subjects with CKD.[13;31] Thus, the process of VSMC abnormal phenotype development may be stimulated in medial wall calcification as well as in atherogenic VC, but this still remains to be proven. Unfortunately, good animal models of medial wall calcification in CKD do not exist. Diffuse medial wall calcification has been observed in MGP-deficient mice.[16] However, the process is so severe and rapid that the model does not lend itself to an analysis of the actions of CKD.

Relationship between Vascular Calcification and Skeletal Remodeling

Clinical observations have suggested a link between VC and skeletal disorders. Epidemiological studies have shown an inverse relationship between bone mineralization and VC. In the Framingham Heart Study, the progression of abdominal aortic calcification correlated with the magnitude of bone loss.[32] A similar relationship has been found in dialysis patients.[3;33] In a cohort of dialysis patients, a strong negative correlation was found between bone mineral density and intimal-media carotid thickness.[33] Another study in CKD patients demonstrated that the severity of VC was greater in patients with hyperphosphatemia, and in those with the adynamic bone disorder compared to high-turnover renal osteodystrophy (ROD).[34] Animal models further confirm this relationship.[10;15;16;25] Thus, vascular calcification can be considered a complication of ROD.

METHODS FOR ASSESSING VASCULAR CALCIFICATION

There are a number of noninvasive methods to measure VC. The two most commonly used to quantify VC are electron-beam computed tomography (EBCT) and multislice (spiral) computed tomography (MSCT) (Figure 3). Both of these techniques allow an accurate assessment of the quantity and progression of calcification, and have significantly facilitated research in this area. They are synchronized with the electrocardiogram (ECG) to acquire cardiac images at a specific point when the heart is at its most quiescent point. Coronary calcium is typically quantified using the Agatston score, which is calculated as the product of the area of the plaque and a density coefficient.[35] A significant limitation with both of these radiological techniques (EBCT and MSCT) is their inability to distinguish between intimal and medial calcification.

Ultrasonography and plain radiographs are semiquantitative techniques that can be used to detect calcification. Both have a relatively low sensitivity, but with wider availability and lower cost they provide a good initial screening tool for the presence of calcification.

The degree of large artery calcification can be indirectly inferred by increases in pulse pressure and pulse wave velocity (PWV). PWV is a reproducible, noninvasive measure of the speed with which the arterial pulse pressure wave (ventricular ejection pressure wave) moves away from the heart.[36] PWV is a reflection of vessel elasticity and increases with arterial stiffening. PWV is a strong predictor of mortality in dialysis patients.[37]

FIGURE 3. MULTISLICE (HELICAL) COMPUTED TOMOGRAM (MSCT) OF THE HEART

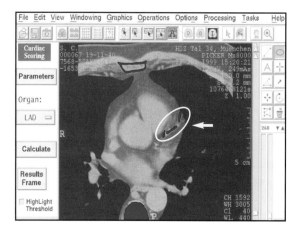

The software is calibrated to color code all tissues of a certain density or higher (usually 120 Hounsfeld Units). In this example, calcified tissue such as vascular calcification of the coronary artery and the bones (spine, sternum, and ribs) are colored blue. The reader then reviews each CT image and circles the region of interest. The software then adds up all of the color coded (i.e. blue) regions in all of the CT slices to achieve the unitless measure of coronary calcification score. The score can be assigned to a specific artery (in this case the left anterior descending); however, the standard coronary artery score is a composite of calcification in all of the major coronary arteries. (From Russell R, Brookshire MA, Zekonis M, and Moe SM. Used with permission).

CLINICAL SIGNIFICANCE OF ARTERIAL CALCIFICATIONS

Both atherogenic and medial calcification can lead to CV disease, but by different mechanisms. In addition, the location of the calcification will dictate the clinical symptoms. However, limitations in imaging techniques do not allow differentiation of atherosclerotic intimal calcification from medial calcification, rendering the identification of the exact mechanism even more arduous. Both coronary and large artery calcification have been clearly associated with increased CV morbidity and mortality in CKD.[5;37;38]

Coronary artery calcification is very common in CKD patients and the magnitude of calcification is markedly higher than in the general population.[3;39] Even young adults on dialysis, with childhood-onset CKD, have a much higher prevalence of coronary calcification than age-matched controls in the general population.[4;40] The intimal calcification that occurs within areas of atherosclerotic plaque may increase plaque fragility, making the vessel wall more vulnerable to shear stresses and more prone to rupture and thrombosis. Though some studies have found coronary calcification a sensitive marker of underlying atherosclerotic disease burden,[41] there is only a moderate correlation between coronary calcification scores by EBCT and the severity of focal stenotic lesions found at angiography in individual lesions.[42] Unfortunately, large outcomes studies in CKD patients with and without coronary artery calcification are lacking. However, in two small studies, the magnitude of coronary artery calcification correlated with mortality in CKD patients on dialysis.[43;44]

In patients without CKD, the severity of coronary calcification does correlate well with outcomes. In patients with known coronary artery disease, coronary calcium scores have been shown to be strong predictor of CV events, independent of the degree of coronary luminal obstruction.[45] The degree of calcification, determined by EBCT, has also been shown to correlate with the prevalence of angina and myocardial infarction.[5] Even in asymptomatic individuals without CKD, coronary artery calcification by EBCT predicted cardiovascular events independent of standard risk factors, and did so more accurately than standard risk factors, C-reactive protein (CRP), and refined Framingham risk stratification.[46]

Diffuse medial wall calcification of the large conduit arteries (e.g., aorta) may influence morbidity and mortality by promoting arterial stiffness and a progressive loss of the cushioning function of blood vessels (arteriosclerosis). The hemodynamic consequences of this condition include an increase in systolic blood pressure (in conjunction with a decrease in diastolic pressure) with a widened pulse pressure, increased PWV, and increased left ventricular afterload. This, in turn, can result in both left ventricular hypertrophy and altered coronary perfusion since the heart has to pump against increased pressure.[47] Studies in the CKD population have demonstrated that VC, independent of age and hypertension, is correlated with increased stiffness in large arteries, higher aortic pulse wave velocity, and left ventricular hypertrophy.[8] In patients on dialysis, aortic stiffness, as measured by PWV, is an independent predictor of all-cause and CV mortality.[48]

Calcification of the cardiac valves may also be a component of the increased CV mortality in CKD. Calcific aortic stenosis is associated with a 50% increase in the risk of death from CV events in nonuremic individuals.[49] CKD patients are much more likely to have mitral and aortic valve calcification than the general population, and the prevalence of valvular calcification has been shown to correlate with the severity of calcium and phosphorus imbalance.[3;50] In a study of peritoneal dialysis patients, the presence of one-or two-valve calcification (demonstrated by echocardiography) increased the probability of all-cause and CV mortality several-fold.[51]

Factors Associated with Arterial Calcifications in Chronic Kidney Disease

A number of factors have been associated with increased severity or prevalence of vascular/valvular calcification in CKD patients (Table 2). Age and duration of dialysis are clearly risk factors for the development of VC.[4;5;8;37] Medial wall calcification is a common finding in diabetes mellitus in the absence of CKD, so it is not surprising that diabetes is also a significant risk factor for calcification in dialysis patients.[5;51]

Some investigators have found an association between hyperphosphatemia and hypercalcemia, and prevalence of VC[4;5;40;51]; however, others have not identified this association.[3;8] The total dose of calcium-based phosphate binder has also been identified as a factor associated with VC.[4;8], and a prospective randomized study found that CKD patients taking the noncalcium binder sevelamer for 1 year were found to have no change in median coronary artery and aortic calcification scores compared to a 28% increase in calcification scores in patients treated with calcium-based binders.[52] Others have recently observed that the contribution of hyperphosphatemia to excess bone resorption is potentially a direct signal stimulating VC.[10] Studies of human vascular smooth muscle cells in vitro confirmed prior observations that extracellular phosphorus is a direct stimulant of altered VSMC phenotype and mineralization. The addition of calcium to these cultures augmented the effect of phosphorus alone.[18] Thus, a direct rela-

TABLE 2. FACTORS ASSOCIATED WITH VASCULAR CALCIFICATION IN CKD PATIENTS

Increasing age
Female gender
White race
Diabetes mellitus
Duration of dialysis therapy
Inflammation
Dyslipidemia and/or increased oxidized LDL
Hyperphosphatemia
High PTH
Low PTH/adynamic bone
Calcium overload
Hypertension
Smoking
Warfarin therapy

Abbreviations: LDL, low-density lipoprotein; PTH, parathyroid hormone.

tionship between ROD and VC through plasma phosphorus appears to be a clinical mechanism of disease that is amenable to careful management, with the potential of preventing the calcific lesions.

The role of PTH as a risk factor for calcification is not clear. A few studies have found a correlation between elevated intact PTH (iPTH) and increased incidence of vascular or valvular calcification.[40;51] Others have not been able to detect an association between VC and iPTH levels.[3;4;8] Low iPTH levels have also been associated with increased calcification.[53] A recent study found that VC was greater in CKD patients with biopsy-proven low osteoblast activity and adynamic bone.[34]

Other factors that have been associated with VC include inflammation (plasma CRP levels or other inflammatory markers),[40;52;54] dyslipidemia,[55;56] and elevated homocysteine levels.[54;55]

Treatment and Prevention

Once calcification has occurred, regression is only rarely observed; therefore, the primary goal of treatment should be prevention and stabilization of existing calcification (Table 3). Preventive measures include control of plasma phosphorus levels, avoiding a positive calcium balance, avoiding oversuppression of parathyroid activity and adynamic bone, glycemic control in diabetic patients, smoking cessation, and measures to minimize inflammation, such as the use of ultrapure dialysate. As previously discussed, warfarin can enhance the potential for VC in CKD patients and, therefore, its use should be minimized.

Elevated plasma phosphorus and calcium, and to a lesser extent PTH, are associated with VC and CV mortality in CKD; thus, normalization should be a priority. However, some data suggest that VC is, at least in part, an iatrogenic phenomenon related to the overuse of calcium-based phosphate binders and vitamin D. This has been the stimulus for the use of new phosphate binders that do not contain calcium, newer vitamin D analogs that may be less calcemic, and the calcimimetic class of compounds for treatment of SHPT (see Chapter 6). These new therapeutics may help reduce the incidence and severity of VC. The use of non–calcium-containing phosphate binders, such as sevelamer or lanthanum carbonate, can reduce the total calcium load, while still effectively controlling phosphorus.[52;57] As described above in a prospective controlled study, sevelamer—along with effective control of phosphorus and calcium—may slow the progression of calcification in CKD patients compared to calcium alone.[51;58;59] It should be noted that patients treated with sevelamer also have a reduction in low-density lipoprotein (LDL) cholesterol. It has yet to be determined whether the attenuation of VC in patients treated with sevelamer is due to its lipid-lowering effect, and/or primarily related to the lower calcium load (with a direct effect on vasculature or indirect effect by impairing bone turnover).

TABLE 3. CLINICAL MEASURES TO STABILIZE OR PREVENT VASCULAR CALCIFICATION IN DIALYSIS PATIENTS

Maintain plasma phosphorus levels between 3.5-5.5 mg/dL (1.13-1.78 mmol/L)
Maintain plasma calcium levels within normal range
Keep calcium-phosphorus product <55 mg^2/dL^2
Keep intact PTH levels between 150-300 pg/mL (16.5-33.0 pmol/L)
Control hypertension
Avoid a positive calcium balance
  • Maintain dialysate calcium concentration at 2.5 mEq/L (1.25 mmol/L)
  • Keep total elemental calcium intake, including binders, <2000 mg/day
Avoiding oversuppression of parathyroid activity and adynamic bone
Maintain good glycemic control in diabetics
Smoking cessation
Measures to minimize inflammation
  • Ultrapure (pyrogen-free) dialysate
Minimize warfarin use

Abbreviation: PTH, parathyroid hormone.

There are several calcification inhibitors, including BMP-7,[10;60] osteopontin,[61] Fetuin A,[62] and teriparatide (PTH 1-34)[63] that are in early developmental stages and may be of clinical benefit in treating ectopic calcification. Teriparatide was recently approved for the treatment of osteoporosis, but has not yet been studied in CKD. Teriparatide has been shown to inhibit osteogenic VC in diabetic mice deficient in LDL receptor.[63] Both BMP-7 and teriparatide are skeletal anabolic agents, and a part of BMP-7's efficacy in VC is mediated by stimulation of bone formation and secondary diminished plasma phosphate concentrations.[10] In addition, there are some data that bisphophosphonates may prevent VC in animal models.[64] However, there are no data from human studies at present with any of these agents.

CONCLUSIONS

The development of VC is an active, cell-mediated process that is widespread in the CKD population and is highly correlated with CV morbidity and mortality. The pathogenesis is complex, involving factors specific to CKD that are currently not well understood. There are few controlled clinical studies in this area and almost none in humans. More research is critical to expand our understanding of the mechanisms of VC and to allow development of effective therapeutic strategies that may prevent or potentially reverse VC.

REFERENCES

1. Longenecker JC, Coresh J, Powe NR, Levey AS, Fink NE, Martin A, Klag MJ: Traditional cardiovascular disease risk factors in dialysis patients compared with the general population: the CHOICE Study. J Am Soc Nephrol 13:1918-1927, 2002

2. Stack AG, Bloembergen WE: Prevalence and clinical correlates of coronary artery disease among new dialysis patients in the United States: a cross-sectional study. J Am Soc Nephrol 12:1516-1523, 2001

3. Braun J, Oldendorf M, Moshage W, Heidler R, Zeitler E, Luft FC: Electron beam computed tomography in the evaluation of cardiac calcification in chronic dialysis patients. Am J Kidney Dis 27:394-401, 1996

*4. Goodman WG, Goldin J, Kuizon BD, Yoon C, Gales B, Sider D, Wang Y, Chung J, Emerick A, Greaser L, Elashoff RM, Salusky IB: Coronary-artery calcification in young adults with end-stage renal disease who are undergoing dialysis. N Engl J Med 342:1478-1483, 2000

*5. Raggi P, Boulay A, Chasan-Taber S, Amin N, Dillon M, Burke SK, Chertow GM: Cardiac calcification in adult hemodialysis patients. A link between end-stage renal disease and cardiovascular disease? J Am Coll Cardiol 39:695-701, 2002

6. Salgueira M, del Toro N, Moreno-Alba R, Jimenez E, Areste N, Palma A: Vascular calcification in the uremic patient: a cardiovascular risk? Kidney Int Suppl S119-S121, 2003

*7. Block GA, Klassen PS, Lazarus JM, Ofsthun N, Lowrie EG, Chertow GM: Mineral metabolism, mortality, and morbidity in maintenance hemodialysis. J Am Soc Nephrol 15:2208-2218, 2004

*8. Guerin AP, London GM, Marchais SJ, Metivier F: Arterial stiffening and vascular calcifications in end-stage renal disease. Nephrol Dial Transplant 15:1014-1021, 2000

*9. Davies MR, Hruska KA: Pathophysiological mechanisms of vascular calcification in end-stage renal disease. Kidney Int 60:472-479, 2001

10. Davies MR, Lund RJ, Mathew S, Hruska KA: Low turnover osteodystrophy and vascular calcification are amenable to skeletal anabolism in an animal model of chronic kidney disease and the metabolic syndrome. J Am Soc Nephrol 16:917-928, 2005

11. Budisavljevic MN, Cheek D, Ploth DW: Calciphylaxis in chronic renal failure. J Am Soc Nephrol 7:978-982, 1996

12. Mazhar AR, Johnson RJ, Gillen D, Stivelman JC, Ryan MJ, Davis CL, Stehman-Breen CO: Risk factors and mortality associated with calciphylaxis in end-stage renal disease. Kidney Int 60:324-332, 2001

13. Moe SM, Duan D, Doehle BP, O'Neill KD, Chen NX: Uremia induces the osteoblast differentiation factor Cbfa1 in human blood vessels. Kidney Int 63:1003-1011, 2003

14. Shanahan CM, Proudfoot D, Tyson KL, Cary NR, Edmonds M, Weissberg PL: Expression of mineralisation-regulating proteins in association with human vascular calcification. Z Kardiol 89 Suppl 2:63-68, 2000

15. Bucay N, Sarosi I, Dunstan CR, Morony S, Tarpley J, Capparelli C, Scully S, Tan HL, Xu W, Lacey DL, Boyle WJ, Simonet WS: osteoprotegerin-deficient mice develop early onset osteoporosis and arterial calcification. Genes Dev 12:1260-1268, 1998

16. Luo G, Ducy P, McKee MD, Pinero GJ, Loyer E, Behringer RR, Karsenty G: Spontaneous calcification of arteries and cartilage in mice lacking matrix GLA protein. Nature 386:78-81, 1997

*17. Reslerova M, Moe SM: Vascular calcification in dialysis patients: pathogenesis and consequences. Am J Kidney Dis 41:S96-S99, 2003

18. Reynolds JL, Joannides AJ, Skepper JN, McNair R, Schurgers LJ, Proudfoot D, Jahnen-Dechent W, Weissberg PL, Shanahan CM: Human vascular smooth muscle cells undergo vesicle-mediated calcification in response to changes in extracellular calcium and phosphate concentrations: a potential mechanism for accelerated vascular calcification in ESRD. J Am Soc Nephrol 15:2857-2867, 2004

*19. Giachelli CM: Vascular calcification mechanisms. J Am Soc Nephrol 15:2959-2964, 2004

20. Jono S, McKee MD, Murry CE, Shioi A, Nishizawa Y, Mori K, Morii H, Giachelli CM: Phosphate regulation of vascular smooth muscle cell calcification. Circ Res 87:E10-E17, 2000

21. Giachelli CM: Vascular calcification: in vitro evidence for the role of inorganic phosphate. J Am Soc Nephrol 14:S300-S304, 2003

22. Chen NX, O'Neill KD, Duan D, Moe SM: Phosphorus and uremic serum up-regulate osteopontin expression in vascular smooth muscle cells. Kidney Int 62:1724-1731, 2002

23. Sweatt A, Sane DC, Hutson SM, Wallin R: Matrix Gla protein (MGP) and bone morphogenetic protein-2 in aortic calcified lesions of aging rats. J Thromb Haemost 1:178-185, 2003

24. Wallin R, Cain D, Sane DC: Matrix Gla protein synthesis and gamma-carboxylation in the aortic vessel wall and proliferating vascular smooth muscle cells—a cell system which resembles the system in bone cells. Thromb Haemost 82:1764-1767, 1999

25. Price PA, Williamson MK, Haba T, Dell RB, Jee WS: Excessive mineralization with growth plate closure in rats on chronic warfarin treatment. Proc Natl Acad Sci U S A 79:7734-7738, 1982

26. Schinke T, Amendt C, Trindl A, Poschke O, Muller-Esterl W, Jahnen-Dechent W: The serum protein alpha2-HS glycoprotein/fetuin inhibits apatite formation in vitro and in mineralizing calvaria cells. A possible role in mineralization and calcium homeostasis. J Biol Chem 271:20789-20796, 1996

27. Schafer C, Heiss A, Schwarz A, Westenfeld R, Ketteler M, Floege J, Muller-Esterl W, Schinke T, Jahnen-Dechent W: The serum protein alpha 2-Heremans-Schmid glycoprotein/fetuin-A is a systemically acting inhibitor of ectopic calcification. J Clin Invest 112:357-366, 2003

*28. Ketteler M, Bongartz P, Westenfeld R, Wildberger JE, Mahnken AH, Bohm R, Metzger T, Wanner C, Jahnen-Dechent W, Floege J: Association of low fetuin-A (AHSG) concentrations in serum with cardiovascular mortality in patients on dialysis: a cross-sectional study. Lancet 361:827-833, 2003

29. Stenvinkel P, Wang K, Qureshi AR, Axelsson J, Pecoits-Filho R, Gao P, Barany P, Lindholm B, Jogestrand T, Heimburger O, Holmes C, Schalling M, Nordfors L: Low fetuin-A levels are associated with cardiovascular death: Impact of variations in the gene encoding fetuin. Kidney Int 67:2383-2392, 2005

30. Wang AY, Woo J, Lam CW, Wang M, Chan IH, Gao P, Lui SF, Li PK, Sanderson JE: Associations of serum fetuin-A with malnutrition, inflammation, atherosclerosis and valvular calcification syndrome and outcome in peritoneal dialysis patients. Nephrol Dial Transplant 20:1676-1685, 2005

*31. Moe SM, Chen NX: Pathophysiology of vascular calcification in chronic kidney disease. Circ Res 95:560-567, 2004

32. Kiel DP, Kauppila LI, Cupples LA, Hannan MT, O'Donnell CJ, Wilson PW: Bone loss and the progression of abdominal aortic calcification over a 25 year period: the Framingham Heart Study. Calcif Tissue Int 68:271-276, 2001

33. Nakashima A, Yorioka N, Tanji C, Asakimori Y, Ago R, Usui K, Shigemoto K, Harada S: Bone mineral density may be related to atherosclerosis in hemodialysis patients. Osteoporos Int 14:369-373, 2003

*34. London GM, Marty C, Marchais SJ, Guerin AP, Metivier F, de Vernejoul MC: Arterial calcifications and bone histomorphometry in end-stage renal disease. J Am Soc Nephrol 15:1943-1951, 2004

35. Agatston AS, Janowitz WR, Hildner FJ, Zusmer NR, Viamonte M, Jr., Detrano R: Quantification of coronary artery calcium using ultrafast computed tomography. J Am Coll Cardiol 15:827-832, 1990

36. London GM: Cardiovascular calcifications in uremic patients: clinical impact on cardiovascular function. J Am Soc Nephrol 14:S305-S309, 2003

37. Blacher J, Guerin AP, Pannier B, Marchais SJ, London GM: Arterial calcifications, arterial stiffness, and cardiovascular risk in end-stage renal disease. Hypertension 38:938-942, 2001

*38. London GM, Guerin AP, Marchais SJ, Metivier F, Pannier B, Adda H: Arterial media calcification in end-stage renal disease: impact on all-cause and cardiovascular mortality. Nephrol Dial Transplant 18:1731-1740, 2003

39. Hujairi NM, Afzali B, Goldsmith DJ: Cardiac calcification in renal patients: what we do and don't know. Am J Kidney Dis 43:234-243, 2004

40. Oh J, Wunsch R, Turzer M, Bahner M, Raggi P, Querfeld U, Mehls O, Schaefer F: Advanced coronary and carotid arteriopathy in young adults with childhood-onset chronic renal failure. Circulation 106:100-105, 2002

41. Sangiorgi G, Rumberger JA, Severson A, Edwards WD, Gregoire J, Fitzpatrick LA, Schwartz RS: Arterial calcification and not lumen stenosis is highly correlated with atherosclerotic plaque burden in humans: a histologic study of 723 coronary artery segments using non-decalcifying methodology. J Am Coll Cardiol 31:126-133, 1998

42. Sharples EJ, Pereira D, Summers S, Cunningham J, Rubens M, Goldsmith D, Yaqoob MM: Coronary artery calcification measured with electron-beam computerized tomography correlates poorly with coronary artery angiography in dialysis patients. Am J Kidney Dis 43:313-319, 2004

43. Matsuoka M, Iseki K, Tamashiro M, Fujimoto N, Higa N, Touma T, Takishita S: Impact of high coronary artery calcification score (CACS) on survival in patients on chronic hemodialysis. Clin Exp Nephrol 8:54-58, 2004

*44. Moe SM, O'Neill KD, Resterova M, Fineberg N, Persohn S, Meyer CA: Natural history of vascular calcification in dialysis and transplant patients. Nephrol Dial Transplant 19:2387-2393, 2004

45. Detrano R, Hsiai T, Wang S, Puentes G, Fallavollita J, Shields P, Stanford W, Wolfkiel C, Georgiou D, Budoff M, Reed J: Prognostic value of coronary calcification and angiographic stenoses in patients undergoing coronary angiography. J Am Coll Cardiol 27:285-290, 1996

46. Arad Y, Goodman KJ, Roth M, Newstein D, Guerci AD: Coronary calcification, coronary disease risk factors, C-reactive protein, and atherosclerotic cardiovascular disease events: the St. Francis Heart Study. J Am Coll Cardiol 46:158-165, 2005

47. London GM: Alterations of arterial function in end-stage renal disease. Nephron 84:111-118, 2000

48. Blacher J, Guerin AP, Pannier B, Marchais SJ, Safar ME, London GM: Impact of aortic stiffness on survival in end-stage renal disease. Circulation 99:2434-2439, 1999

49. Otto CM, Lind BK, Kitzman DW, Gersh BJ, Siscovick DS: Association of aortic-valve sclerosis with cardiovascular mortality and morbidity in the elderly. N Engl J Med 341:142-147, 1999

50. Rufino M, Garcia S, Jimenez A, Alvarez A, Miquel R, Delgado P, Marrero D, Torres A, Hernandez D, Lorenzo V: Heart valve calcification and calcium x phosphorus product in hemodialysis patients: analysis of optimum values for its prevention. Kidney Int Suppl S115-S118, 2003

*51. Wang AY, Wang M, Woo J, Lam CW, Li PK, Lui SF, Sanderson JE: Cardiac valve calcification as an important predictor for all-cause mortality and cardiovascular mortality in long-term peritoneal dialysis patients: a prospective study. J Am Soc Nephrol 14:159-168, 2003

52. Chertow GM, Raggi P, McCarthy JT, Schulman G, Silberzweig J, Kuhlik A, Goodman WG, Boulay A, Burke SK, Toto RD: The effects of sevelamer and calcium acetate on proxies of atherosclerotic and arteriosclerotic vascular disease in hemodialysis patients. Am J Nephrol 23:307-314, 2003

53. Ahmed S, O'Neill KD, Hood AF, Evan AP, Moe SM: Calciphylaxis is associated with hyperphosphatemia and increased osteopontin expression by vascular smooth muscle cells. Am J Kidney Dis 37:1267-1276, 2001

54. Stompor T, Pasowicz M, Sullowicz W, Dembinska-Kiec A, Janda K, Wojcik K, Tracz W, Zdzienicka A, Klimeczek P, Janusz-Grzybowska E: An association between coronary artery calcification score, lipid profile, and selected markers of chronic inflammation in ESRD patients treated with peritoneal dialysis. Am J Kidney Dis 41:203-211, 2003

55. Kronenberg F, Mundle M, Langle M, Neyer U: Prevalence and progression of peripheral arterial calcifications in patients with ESRD. Am J Kidney Dis 41:140-148, 2003

56. Tamashiro M, Iseki K, Sunagawa O, Inoue T, Higa S, Afuso H, Fukiyama K: Significant association between the progression of coronary artery calcification and dyslipidemia in patients on chronic hemodialysis. Am J Kidney Dis 38:64-69, 2001

57. D'Haese PC, Spasovski GB, Sikole A, Hutchison A, Freemont TJ, Sulkova S, Swanepoel C, Pejanovic S, Djukanovic L, Balducci A, Coen G, Sulowicz W, Ferreira A, Torres A, Curic S, Popovic M, Dimkovic N, De Broe ME: A multicenter study on the effects of lanthanum carbonate (Fosrenol) and calcium carbonate on renal bone disease in dialysis patients. Kidney Int Suppl S73-S78, 2003

*58. Chertow GM, Burke SK, Raggi P: Sevelamer attenuates the progression of coronary and aortic calcification in hemodialysis patients. Kidney Int 62:245-252, 2002

59. Raggi P, Bommer J, Chertow GM: Valvular calcification in hemodialysis patients randomized to calcium-based phosphorus binders or sevelamer. J Heart Valve Dis 13:134-141, 2004

*60. Davies MR, Lund RJ, Hruska KA: BMP-7 is an efficacious treatment of vascular calcification in a murine model of atherosclerosis and chronic renal failure. J Am Soc Nephrol 14:1559-1567, 2003

61. Steitz SA, Speer MY, McKee MD, Liaw L, Almeida M, Yang H, Giachelli CM: Osteopontin inhibits mineral deposition and promotes regression of ectopic calcification. Am J Pathol 161:2035-2046, 2002

62. Jahnen-Dechent W, Schafer C, Heiss A, Grotzinger J: Systemic inhibition of spontaneous calcification by the serum protein alpha 2-HS glycoprotein/fetuin. Z Kardiol 90 Suppl 3:47-56, 2001

63. Shao JS, Cheng SL, Charlton-Kachigian N, Loewy AP, Towler DA: Teriparatide (human parathyroid hormone (1-34)) inhibits osteogenic vascular calcification in diabetic low density lipoprotein receptor-deficient mice. J Biol Chem 278:50195-50202, 2003

64. Price PA, Faus SA, Williamson MK: Bisphosphonates alendronate and ibandronate inhibit artery calcification at doses comparable to those that inhibit bone resorption. Arterioscler Thromb Vasc Biol 21:817-824, 2001

*Suggested Reading

6

TREATMENT
APPROACHES
IN CKD

Tilman B. Drüeke
Sharon M. Moe
Craig B. Langman

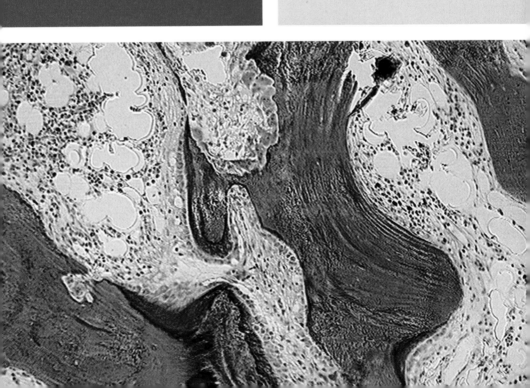

CHAPTER 6

TREATMENT APPROACHES IN CKD

Tilman B. Drüeke, Sharon M. Moe, Craig B. Langman

The treatment modalities for renal bone disease are designed to normalize phosphorus and calcium, and to optimize parathyroid hormone (PTH) levels, while improving bone strength and minimizing extraskeletal complications. In order to minimize the severity of renal osteodystrophy (ROD), it is important to consider the control of all three components of the management strategy: calcium, phosphorus, and PTH. The primary treatment considerations for accomplishing these goals include:

1. Restriction of dietary phosphate intake commensurate with stage of CKD

2. Optimizing kidney replacement therapy

3. Administration of dietary phosphate binders

4. Administration of oral calcium supplements

5. Administration of vitamin D or its derivatives

6. Administration of calcimimetics

7. Parathyroidectomy

Over the last decade, many of the original therapeutic approaches to ROD have been critically examined and revised. Hypocalcemia, hyperphosphatemia, and secondary hyperparathyroidism (SHPT) have been aggressively treated with calcium supplements, calcium-based phosphate binders, and calcitriol. While this approach is effective in many patients, it is now recognized that it can result in a maldistribution of delivered calcium and phosphorus load, with consequent vascular and soft-tissue calcifications, and increased mortality.[1] With the increased use of calcium and calcitriol, the frequency of high-turnover bone disease from SHPT has been reduced. However, this reduction has been accompanied by an increase in the prevalence of adynamic (low-turnover) bone disease, which is associated with both increased fractures and vascular calcification.[2-4] These findings have led to the revision of target ranges for phosphorus, calcium, and PTH (see Appendix), specific to each stage of CKD. It also has led to the awareness that alternative pharmacological approaches were needed for the treatment of renal bone disease, which in turn led to the development of new oral phosphate binders, vitamin D analogs, and a new therapeutic class, calcimimetics. The potential ability of daily and nocturnal hemodialysis regimens to improve mineral imbalances is yet another intriguing new development in this area.[5]

SPECTRUM OF BONE AND MINERAL DISEASE IN CKD

Disturbances in calcium, phosphorus, and vitamin D metabolism occur early in CKD and eventually lead to SHPT. The cascade of pathophysiological events in CKD that lead to these bone and mineral disorders include[6;7]:

- *diminished kidney function*, leading to reduced phosphorus excretion and subsequent phosphorus retention;

- *elevated plasma phosphorus*, causing direct suppression of calcitriol production;

- *decreased ability of the kidneys* to convert minimally active calcidiol [25(OH)D] to active D hormone (calcitriol) as a result of a reduction in functional kidney mass;

- *decreased calcitriol production*, leading to reduced calcium absorption from the intestines and contributing to hypocalcemia, which is enhanced by hyperphosphatemia;

- *hypocalcemia, reduced calcitriol synthesis, and elevated plasma phosphorus levels*, stimulating the production and secretion of PTH, and increasing parathyroid cell mass by both hypertrophy and hyperplasia, resulting in SHPT; and

- *sustained elevation of PTH levels (SHPT)* with increased osteoblast and osteoclast activity, resulting in high bone turnover.

These alterations in bone and mineral balance begin to occur once the GFR has dropped below 70 ml/min/1.73 m^2.[6;8] Therefore, the K/DOQI Clinical Practice Guidelines for CKD recommend that all adult patients with GFR <60 mL/min/1.73 m^2 (Stages 3 and 4 CKD) should be evaluated for bone disease and disorders of calcium and phosphorus metabolism.[9] The primary bone lesion seen in patients with moderate loss of kidney function is osteitis fibrosa related to hyperparathyroidism and high bone turnover, although some patients in this group may have histological evidence of low turnover/adynamic bone disease.[10] Children may manifest bone disease in Stage 2 CKD, perhaps related to their growth rate and bone turnover.

As kidney disease progresses, bone and mineral metabolism imbalances increase in severity. Nearly all patients with kidney failure have histological evidence of ROD at the initiation of dialysis.[11] However, in CKD Stage 5, the prevalence of the various forms of ROD appears to be changing. Histological studies have found an increasing incidence of adynamic bone disease and a decreasing rate of osteitis fibrosa.[12] This may be due partially to a changing patient population—such as increased prevalence of diabetic and elderly patients—but it also may reflect protocols for the treatment of ROD used during the last 10-15 years. Adynamic bone disease has been associated with high-dose calcium-containing binder use, treatment with large doses of active vitamin D sterols, and consequent relatively low PTH levels.[4] Both sustained high or low levels of PTH can negatively impact bone metabolism and have been linked to increased fracture rates.[13;14] It is also possible that the loss of mineral buffering potential that occurs with low bone turnover may be a risk factor for extraskeletal deposition of calcium .[15]

Pathological vascular and soft-tissue calcification is another critical element of the altered bone and mineral metabolism in CKD. Increased plasma phosphorus, calcium, and calcium-phosphorus product (CaXP), as well as an increased calcium load, have all been linked to cardiovascular abnormalities and increased mortality in CKD.[16-19]

Ongoing monitoring and treatment adjustments to maintain calcium, phosphorus, and PTH within the target levels (see Appendix) are critical to minimizing ROD, vascular calcification, and mortality in CKD. Early intervention to keep CKD patients within the suggested target ranges in CKD Stages 3-4 may pre-empt the progression and severity of bone disease. It is often difficult to balance simultaneous assessment and treatment of phosphorus, calcium, and PTH abnormalities in clinical practice. In addition, these values can fluctuate, and thus it is trends—rather than single measurements—that should be followed carefully. To maximize clinical outcomes, a diligent effort should be made to achieve the K/DOQI target ranges for calcium, phosphorus, and PTH in each patient, but this may not be possible in every patient or achieved with complete consistency in many patients. The K/DOQI target ranges are meant to be goals for adequate care, but managing bone and mineral imbalances in CKD is complex, and in some cases one element may need to be prioritized over another. The morbidity and mortality data presented in Chapter 4 are valuable in making informed clinical decisions about the management of ROD.

The following is a review of the various treatment strategies currently recommended to correct bone and mineral imbalances in CKD.

RENAL REPLACEMENT THERAPY

Increased-frequency renal replacement therapy is an important treatment consideration in managing mineral balance and bone disease. This includes adapting the dialysate and renal prescription based on individual patient needs. The dialysis technique (daily, nocturnal, diafiltration, or continuous) is also an important consideration in managing mineral balance.

Phosphate

The removal of phosphate during dialysis is mediated by diffusive and convective clearance. The total quantity of phosphate removed depends on plasma phosphorus concentration at initiation of dialysis, ultrafiltration rate, dialyzer surface area, and frequency and duration of dialysis.

The typical 4-hour hemodialysis session, performed three times per week, is inadequate to maintain a net zero balance between phosphorus intake and output. Approximately 30 mmol (400 mg) of phosphate is removed during a typical, 4-hour, high-flux hemodialysis session.[20] Assuming a 700 mg per day dietary phosphorus absorption, there is still a net positive phosphorus balance of 3,700 mg per week, which requires large quantities of phosphate binders to effect a neutral balance. A dialysis prescription that increases phosphate removal would be of clinical importance.

It had been generally accepted that the majority of phosphate removal occurs early in the dialysis session, with an initial rapid fall in plasma phosphorus, followed by a slow equilibration from the intracellular compartment that leads to a low plasma-to-dialysate gradient and a slowing of mass transfer of phosphate as the dialysis period proceeds.[21;22] Several studies have demonstrated that even though a major fraction of phosphate is removed during the first hour, there is a significant and relatively constant removal of phosphate throughout the duration of dialysis.[20;23] This is supported by clinical studies showing that long-term nocturnal dialysis is able to maintain normal plasma phosphorus levels without the need for binders, and that long-duration, slow-flow nocturnal dialysis is better able to control phosphorus than short-duration, high-efficiency daily dialysis.[5;24]

Calcium

The K/DOQI Guidelines for Bone Metabolism and Disease in CKD recommend that the standard dialysate calcium concentration for both hemodialysis and peritoneal dialysis should be 2.5 mEq/L (1.25 mM).[25] At this concentration, there should be minimal net movement of calcium to or from the patient, although recent studies with long-term daily dialysis found that patients dialyzed with a 2.5 mEq/L dialysate solution required calcium supplementation to maintain plasma calcium levels.[5]

A lower dialysate calcium concentration (1.5-2.0 mEq/L) will result in a net movement of calcium out of the plasma and may be beneficial for patients with elevated plasma calcium level, keeping in mind that reduced calcium intake may exacerbate SHPT. Indeed, lower dialysate calcium concentration may be beneficial for those patients with adynamic bone disease [iPTH <100 pg/mL (11 pmol/L)] by raising plasma PTH levels. Calcium dialysate concentrations of 3.5 mEq/L (1.75 mM) may be appropriate for patients with hypocalcemia and those who do not require phosphate binders or vitamin D analogs. However, the net change in calcium balance as a result of changes in dialysate calcium concentration is minimal compared to changes from diet or calcium-containing phosphate binders. In patients treated with calcimimetics, it may be necessary to increase the dialysate calcium concentration. Also, when determining a calcium dialysate concentration, it should be kept in mind that growing children require a positive calcium balance.

Preliminary studies have indicated that daily nocturnal hemodialysis may offer significant advantages in maintaining nutritional homeostasis, including normal bone mineral balance, without phosphate binders and/or vitamin D supplementation.[5;26;27] While these results are promising, there is still limited long-term experience and further analysis is needed to assess patient acceptance and overall costs.

CONTROL OF PHOSPHORUS

Typically, dietary phosphorus intake ranges from 800-1,400 mg (25-44 mmol) per day. In healthy adults, plasma phosphorus levels are maintained within a narrow range, approximately 2.5-4.5 mg/dL (0.8 -1.4 mmol/L).* Kidney excretion is the primary mechanism for control of phosphorus homeostasis. Approximately 30% of ingested phosphorus is excreted directly through the gastrointestinal tract while the rest is absorbed and excreted by the kidneys.

As kidney function declines in CKD, the ability to maintain phosphorus homeostasis is compromised. As an initial compensatory mechanism to maintain phosphorus levels, there is a decrease in the rate of renal tubular reabsorption, which is partially mediated by PTH. This often allows phosphorus levels to be maintained within the normal range until GFR falls below 20-25 mL/min/1.73 m^2 (CKD Stages 3-4). At this point, kidney excretion cannot quantitatively eliminate sufficient phosphorus derived from the diet, and hyperphosphatemia ensues. This tendency for hyperphosphatemia worsens as kidney function diminishes further.

* Note: See the distinction between the terms "phosphorus" and "phosphate" in Chapter 3

When dialysis is initiated, phosphorus is removed in the dialysate; however, with a standard dialysis regimen, this clearance is inadequate to maintain a net zero phosphorus balance in the majority of patients. Therefore, dietary absorption of phosphorus must be reduced. This is accomplished through dietary restrictions, plus the addition of oral phosphate binders, which reduce absorption and increase gastrointestinal elimination of ingested phosphate. Reduction of dietary phosphorus intake is of critical importance in maintaining phosphorus levels. There are several excellent resources on dietary considerations to control phosphorus intake.[28-30] The focus in this chapter will be on therapeutic use of phosphate binders.

Hyperphosphatemia is prevalent in the population with CKD Stages 4-5. A recent retrospective analysis of over 6,000 patients in the U.S. found that 70% of patients had phosphorus concentrations >5.0 mg/dL (1.6 mmol/L), 39% had levels >6.5 mg/dL (2.08 mmol/L), and 10% had levels >9.0 mg/dL (2.88 mmol/L). Hyperphosphatemia is associated with a variety of calcific complications and increased mortality.[17;31] The K/DOQI Guidelines for Bone and Mineral Metabolism in CKD recommend maintaining plasma phosphorus levels in the range of 1.1-1.8 mmol/L (3.5-5.5 mg/dL) and the CaXP below (55 mg^2/dL^2) 4.44 mmol^2/L^2.[25]

Until the mid-1980s, aluminum-based oral phosphate binders were the primary agents used to control phosphorus absorption. While very effective in binding phosphorus, aluminum is itself largely eliminated by the kidney. Therefore, many CKD patients treated with aluminum-based binders developed significant accumulation of aluminum, with associated toxic side-effects, including aluminum bone disease (osteomalacia) and encephalopathy.[32] With the recognition of the toxic effects of aluminum, there was a shift in the 1980s to calcium-based binders (calcium carbonate and calcium acetate). Calcium-based binders can effectively reduce plasma phosphorus levels. However, it has recently become clear that excess calcium salts, particularly in the presence of elevated phosphorus levels, can lead to calcium deposition in soft tissues.[33] The use of large doses of calcium-based binders is associated with increased risk for hypercalcemia, metastatic calcifications,[34] and coronary artery calcifications.[18;19] The K/DOQI Clinical Practice Guidelines for Bone Metabolism and Disease in CKD recommend that the total dose of elemental calcium provided by calcium-based phosphate binders should not exceed 1,500 mg/day, with the total calcium intake per day from diet and binders to not exceed 2,000 mg (Table 1). This suggested value for maximum calcium intake was based on the Institute of Medicine's recommendation of 2,500 mg/day as an upper limit in normal adults, with consideration of the reduced kidney excretion of calcium in CKD. Calcium-based binders should also be avoided in dialysis patients who have a corrected plasma calcium level >10.2 mg/dL (2.55 mmol/L) or whose iPTH level is <150 pg/mL (16.5 pmol/L).[25] Calcium citrate should be avoided in CKD, as citrate leads to increased aluminum absorption.[25]

This concern about the side-effects of both calcium- and aluminum-based phosphate binders for CKD has stimulated the development of new calcium- and aluminum-free binders. Sevelamer hydrochloride (RenaGel®) is a calcium-free, aluminum-free phosphate binder that was introduced in 1998. It is a large-molecular-weight resin that is not absorbed by the intestine. Its phosphate-binding capacity is roughly equivalent to that of calcium carbonate. The effectiveness of sevelamer in controlling hyperphosphatemia is well demonstrated.[35;36] Sevelamer has minimal effect on plasma calcium levels, resulting in a reduction in CaXP. In

TABLE 1. CALCIUM CONTENT OF COMMON CALCIUM-BASED PHOSPHATE BINDERS

Compound	Brand Name	Compound Content (mg)	Elemental Calcium (mg)	# of pills to provide 1,500 mg elemental calcium*
Calcium Acetate	Phoslo®	667	167	9
	Chooz™ (Gum) TUMS™ (Regular)	500 mg	200 mg	7.5
	TUMS EX™	750 mg	300 mg	5
	TUMS Ultra™	1,000 mg	400 mg	3.75
	LiquiCal	1,200 mg	480 mg	3
Calcium Carbonate	CalciChew™ CalciMix™ Oscal 500™ TUMS 500™	1,250 mg	500 mg	3
	Caltrate 600™ NephroCalci™	1,500 mg	600 mg	2.5
Calcium Citrate	Citra-Cal®			Not Recommended
	MagneBind® 200	450 Ca acetate/ 200 Mg Carb	113 (Mg = 57)	13
Calcium Acetate/ Magnesium Carbonate	MagneBind®	300 Ca acetate/ 300 Mg Carb	76 (Mg = 85)	20

*Maximum recommended daily calcium intake from K/DOQI Guidelines for Bone Metabolism and Disease in CKD.[25]

addition to its phosphate-binding properties, several studies have shown that sevelamer reduces total and low-density lipoprotein (LDL) cholesterol, and increases HDL cholesterol in either healthy patients or those on dialysis.[37] In a randomized comparative trial, it was demonstrated that the long-term (1-year) administration of sevelamer to chronic hemodialysis patients led to fewer episodes of hypercalcemia, improved control of SHPT, and slowed the progression—or even arrested—coronary artery and aortic calcifications, compared to the administration of calcium carbonate or calcium acetate.[38] One safety consideration with sevelamer hydrochloride is its potential to decrease plasma bicarbonate levels and therefore exacerbate metabolic acidosis.[39;40]

Lanthanum carbonate (Fosrenol™) is another calcium- and aluminum-free phosphate binder that has recently been approved for commercial use. Lanthanum has a high phosphate-binding capacity and clinical trials have established its effectiveness in controlling hyperphosphatemia.[41;42] Lanthanum is also chewable, offering an alternative for patients with swallowing difficulties. Lanthanum appears to be poorly absorbed in the intestine and has been administered in controlled clinical studies for up to 5 years in a few patients without histological signs of bone toxicity, such as aluminum-associated bone disease[41]. However, since it has been shown to accumulate (primarily in the liver) in animal studies when given in high amounts, potential long-term toxicity cannot be firmly excluded at this time.[43]

Aluminum-containing phosphate binders may be considered in some treatment-resistant cases, but only for short time periods (less than 4 weeks). Low doses (2 g/day) of magnesium hydroxide or carbonate can be used in place of, or in association with, calcium salts for the control of plasma phosphate. Low-dose magnesium treatment is accompanied by only slight increases in plasma magnesium concentration when used with a simultaneous decrease in dialysate magnesium concentration, and does not appear to have any long-term deleterious effects on bone mineralization. However, there are very limited studies of magnesium-based binder use. Higher doses should not be used, in general, since they frequently lead to diarrhea and favor the occurrence of hyperkalemia.

In summary (Table 2), calcium-based phosphate binders can be used as a primary therapy in patients who: are not prone to hypercalcemia; have no clinical or radiological evidence of soft tissue calcification; or have PTH levels persistently higher than 150 pg/mL (16.5 pmol/L). In all other patients with hyperphosphatemia, calcium-free compounds should be used as the initial, preferred therapy. In some instances, a combination of calcium and non–calcium-based binders can be used. Calcium acetate (PhosLo®) salts have the advantage of higher phosphate-binding capacity than calcium carbonate salts; therefore, less total elemental calcium is required for phosphorus binding, with reduced calcium exposure and absorption.[44]

Every effort should be made to help the patient control their phosphorus intake without jeopardizing their nutritional status. The renal dietitian plays a critical role in this process of educating and motivating CKD patients on dietary compliance.

TABLE 2. SUMMARY OF CLINICALLY USEFUL PHOSPHATE BINDERS

Phosphate Binder	Common Product Name	Advantages	Potential Side Effects/Disadvantages
Aluminum- based	Aluminum Hydroxides: Amphojel® Alu-Caps® Alu-Tabs® AltenaGEL® Dialume® Aluminum Carbonate: Basojel® Carafate®	High phosphate binding capacity. Does not add to calcium load. Inexpensive Readily accessible	High potential for aluminum toxicity and bone mineral defects with long term use Constipation GI Distress Chalky taste
Calcium carbonate	Tums® Oscal® Calcichew® Caltrate® Calci-mix® Titralac® Chooz gum®	Inexpensive Readily accessible	Hypercalcemia Extraskeletal calcification Constipation
Calcium acetate	PhosLo®	Higher phosphate binding capacity and less calcium absorption than calcium carbonate	Hypercalcemia Extraskeletal calcification Constipation
Magnesium-based	MagneBind® (Magnesium carbonate and calcium carbonate combination)	Less total calcium load	Diarrhea, Potential for magnesium toxicity. Potential for hyperkalemia.
Sevelamer	RenaGel®	Does not add to calcium load Demonstrated to reduce the risk of cardiovascular calcification Reduces cholesterol levels	Requires large doses/pill size which may effect patient compliance. Decreases bicarbonate possibly enhancing metabolic acidosis. Potentially effects absorption of lipid soluble vitamins GI Distress Expensive
Lanthanum	Fosrenal®	Does not add to calcium load	Potential for accumulation of lanthanum in bone

VITAMIN D AND ITS DERIVATIVES

The hormonal vitamin D system requires the participation of three different organs in the body for activation. First, the parent compound vitamin D is manufactured by the action of the sun in the skin and is absorbed from dietary sources. Vitamin D [ergocalciferol (D_2) or cholecalciferol (D_3)] is metabolically inactive and requires sequential hydroxylations to become biologically active. The first step in the metabolic activation of vitamin D is hydroxylation of the 25 carbon in the liver to form 25-hydroxyvitamin D [25(OH)D]. This hepatic hydroxylation is minimally regulated, so that the levels of 25(OH)D are proportional to vitamin D intake, and are therefore a good measure of vitamin D nutritional status. The second, and more tightly regulated, step is hydroxylation in the 1α position to form the active vitamin D hormone, $1\alpha,25$-dihydroxyvitamin D [$1,25(OH)_2D$]. This conversion occurs almost exclusively in the proximal tubule of the kidney due to the action of the renal enzyme, $25(OH)D-1\alpha$-hydroxylase. The availability of 1α-hydroxylase, and therefore the rate of active D hormone production, is tightly controlled.

In its active form, $1,25(OH)_2D$ is able to bind to vitamin D receptors (VDR) and modulate transcription activities in the target organs. The primary target organs for $1,25(OH)_2D$ are the intestines, parathyroid gland, bone, and kidneys. $1,25(OH)_2D$ interacts with intestinal VDR, to stimulate the transport of dietary calcium from the intestinal lumen. In the parathyroid gland, $1,25(OH)_2D$, as part of a hormonal feedback mechanism, has a direct suppressive effect on PTH synthesis. Stimulation of VDR in the kidney results in decreased 1α-hydroxylase activity and increased kidney reabsorption of calcium and phosphorus. In addition to the primary target organs, VDRs are located throughout the body and play a role in a diverse group of physiological functions, including maturation of skin and hematopoietic cells, immune function, and production and release of insulin.[45]

Hyperphosphatemia directly suppresses 1α-hydroxylase activity in the kidney. As CKD progresses, the ability to produce $1,25(OH)_2D$ diminishes, resulting in reduced calcium absorption and hypocalcemia. The hypocalcemia and reduced levels of $1,25(OH)_2D$ lead to SHPT. If this cascade of events continues unchecked, the parathyroid gland will hypertrophy, and eventually develop nodular hyperplasia. In such circumstances, reduced VDR expression occurs. This reduction may be irreversible, leading to an inability of $1,25(OH)_2D$ to suppress SHPT.

Vitamin D repletion is an important therapeutic consideration in treating both hypocalcemia and SHPT in CKD. The benefit of vitamin D therapy on elevated PTH has been well established, and several studies have demonstrated improved bone metabolism and density with active D sterol therapy.[10;46;47] However, in addition to these beneficial affects, active D sterols stimulate the intestinal absorption of calcium and phosphorus, which can cause hyperphosphatemia, elevate CaXP, and add to the total calcium load. Another potential complication with vitamin D therapy is oversuppression of the parathyroid gland, leading to adynamic bone disease.[48] Patients with SHPT should be monitored closely, and any treatment decisions on D hormone therapy need to take into account the patient's plasma phosphorus, calcium, and PTH levels.

In CKD Stages 3 and 4

Stage 3 or 4 CKD patients retain some 1α-hydroxylase activity and are therefore frequently able to produce adequate levels of $1,25(OH)_2D$, if they are not deficient in 25(OH)D. Unfortunately, the majority of CKD Stage 3 and 4 patients have either vitamin D insufficiency [defined as plasma 25(OH)D levels between 16-30 ng/mL (40-75 nmol/L)] or vitamin D deficiency [defined as plasma 25(OH)D levels below 16 ng/mL (40 nmol/L)].[49;50] The first step in treating elevated PTH in these patients is to ensure that 25(OH)D levels are in the upper limit of normal. This can usually be accomplished by supplementation with ergocalciferol or cholecalciferol. If plasma 25(OH)D levels are greater than 30 ng/mL (75 nmol/L) and PTH levels remain elevated, treatment with active D sterols (alfacalcidol, calcitriol, or doxercalciferol) should be considered (see Algorithms 1 and 2).

ALGORITHM 1. VITAMIN D SUPPLEMENTATION IN CKD (STAGES 3-4) [25]

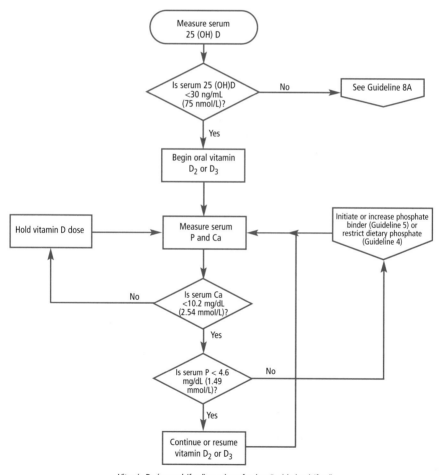

In CKD patients with serum P <4.6 mg/dL (1.49 mmol/L), serum Ca <9.5 mg/dL (2.37 mmol/L), and serum PTH in the higher level of the target range for CKD stage (Stage 3: 35-70 pg/mL [3.85-7.7 pmol/L]; Stage 4: 70-110 pg/mL [7.7-12.1 pmol/L]

Vitamin D$_2$ (ergocalciferol) may be safer than D$_3$ (cholecalciferol).
When the 25(OH)D level is < 15 ng/ml (37 nmol/L), 50,000 IU weekly for 4 doses followed by monthly for 4 doses is effective. With 25(OH)D levels of 20-30 ng/mL (50-75 nmol/L), 50,000 IU monthly for 6 months is recommended.

ALGORITHM 2. MANAGEMENT OF CKD PATIENTS (STAGES 3-4) WITH ACTIVE VITAMIN D STEROLS[25]

In CKD patients, Stages 3 and 4, with stable renal function, compliant with visits and medications with serum phosphorus levels < 4.6 mg/dL (1.49 mmol/L), calcium < 9.5 mg/dL (2.37 mmol/L), and 25(OH)D ≥ 30 ng/mL (75 nmol/L)

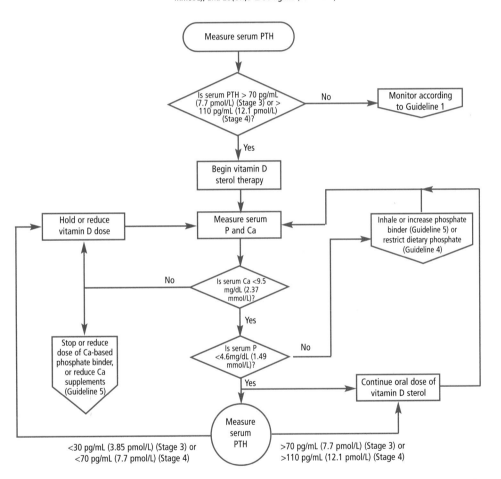

Oral active vitamin D sterols available include calcitrol, alfacalcidol, and doxercalciferol; calcitrol (USA, Canada) and alfacalcidol (Canada and Europe) are approved for use in CKD, Stages 3 and 4. Initial doses should be low (calcitrol 0.25 µg/day or alfacalcidol, 0.25 µg/day). The dose of calcitrol should rarely exceed 0.5 µg/day and then only if the corrected levels of calcium increase by less than 0.2-0.3 mg/dL.

In CKD Stage 5

There is little or no kidney 1α-hydroxylase activity left in Stage 5 CKD. Treatment of patients with significant hyperparathyroidism or hypocalcemia requires vitamin D sterols that are either active on administration or that only require hepatic C_{25} hydroxylation. The initiation and maintenance of vitamin D therapy needs to be based not just on plasma PTH levels, but also plasma phosphorus and plasma ionized (or corrected total) calcium concentrations (see Algorithms 3, 4, and 5).[25]

ALGORITHM 3. MANAGING VITAMIN D STEROLS BASED ON PLASMA CALCIUM LEVELS[25]

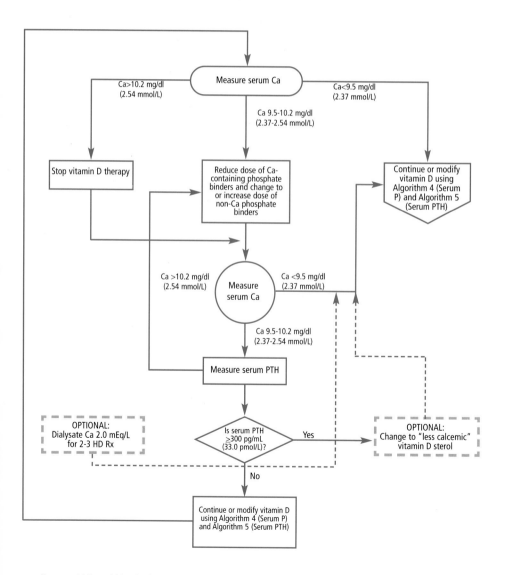

ALGORITHM 4. MANAGING VITAMIN D STEROLS BASED ON PLASMA PHOSPHORUS LEVELS[25]

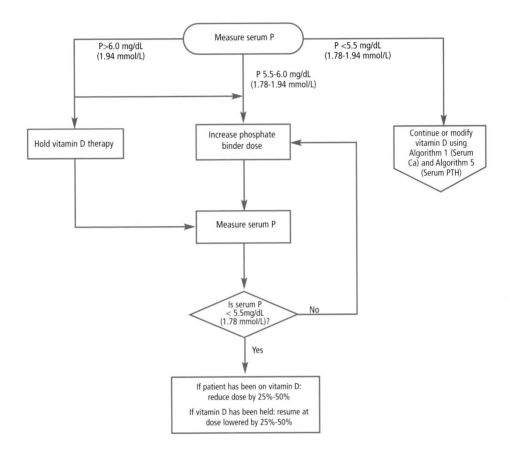

ALGORITHM 5. MANAGING VITAMIN D STEROLS BASED ON INTACT PTH LEVELS[25]

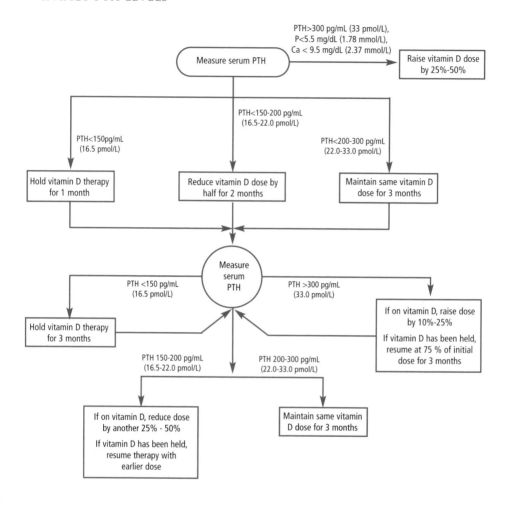

When intact serum PTH is between 300-500 pg/mL (33.0 - 55.0 pmol/L) and changes on two successive determinations are small (<25%), there is no need to modify vitamin D dose as long as P and Ca are within the desired limits (see Algorithms 3 and 4).

When intact PTH is persistently >500-800 pg/mL (55.0 -88.0 pmol/L) and P is 5.5-6.5 mg/dL (1.78-1.94 mmol/L) and/or Ca is 10.2-10.5 mg/dL (2.54-2.62 mmol/L), a trial with a "less calcemic" analog may be warranted for 3-5 months; if such a patient fails to respond, parathyroidectomy may be required.

Alfacalcidol and calcitriol have been extensively used since the 1970s to treat hypocalcemia and SHPT in Stage 5 CKD. They are effective in reducing PTH, but they have a narrow therapeutic window, such that they easily induce hypercalcemia and elevations in plasma phosphorus. There has been extensive research to develop vitamin D analogs that can selectively reduce PTH while minimizing increases in plasma calcium and phosphorus levels. Recently introduced vitamin D analogs include 22-oxa-calcitriol (maxacalcitol), 19-nor-1,25(OH)$_2$ vitamin D2 (paricalcitol), and 1α-(OH) vitamin D$_2$ (doxercalciferol). In the experimental setting, this new generation of vitamin D analogs has considerable therapeutic potential, because of their lower calcemic activity. Unfortunately, in the routine clinical setting—while they are all efficacious in reducing PTH—none has been shown to have entirely lost the capacity of inducing an increase in plasma calcium or phosphate, and none has as yet been demonstrated to be superior to calcitriol or alfacalcidol in controlling SHPT.

In hemodialysis patients, active vitamin D compounds can be administered orally or intravenously. Oral administration can be done on a daily basis or as an intermittent bolus dose (1-4 times per week). Intravenous dose is given as an intermittent dose (3 times per week with dialysis). There is some evidence that intravenous and/or intermittent dosing may be preferable, but the route and mode of administration of vitamin D is probably of minimal significance in the majority of patients.[51;52]

Currently available vitamin D therapies are shown in Table 3 and reviewed next.

VITAMIN D PRODUCTS

Calcitriol
Calcitriol, 1,25(OH)$_2$D$_3$, is the naturally occurring form of vitamin D hormone. It has a long history of clinical use in the treatment of hypocalcemia and SHPT, both as an oral and intravenous agent in CKD Stages 3-5.

Alfacalcidol
Alfacalcidol (1α-hydroxyvitamin D$_3$) is a prohormone that needs to be C$_{25}$ hydroxylated in the liver to 1,25(OH)$_2$D$_3$ before it has significant activity on VDR. It has been used successfully to manage renal bone disease since the 1970s. Controlled clinical trials have demonstrated its effectiveness for both intravenous and oral administration in hemodialysis and as an oral therapy in CKD Stages 3-4.[10;53;54]

Dihydrotachysterol
Dihydrotachysterol$_2$ (DHT$_2$) is hydroxylated *in vivo* to 25(OH)DHT$_2$ and 1,25(OH)$_2$DHT$_2$. DHT was one of the first vitamin D derivatives used to treat renal bone disease, but there are few well-documented reports on its efficacy and safety.[55;56] DHT is available in both tablet and liquid form for oral administration only.

Paricalcitol
Paricalcitol [19-nor-1,25(OH)$_2$ vitamin D$_2$] is a sterol derived from vitamin D$_2$ that lacks the carbon-19 methylene group found in all natural vitamin D metabolites. Intravenous paricalcitol has

TABLE 3. SUMMARY OF CLINICALLY USEFUL VITAMIN D PRODUCTS FOR CKD

Compound	Formulation	Brand Name	*Initial Dose (micrograms)	Comments
Alfacalcidol $1\alpha(OH)D_3$	Oral	Alpha-D3® (Teva Pharmaceuticals) One-Alpha® (Leo Pharma) Alfarol® (Chugai)	1.75-7.0 per week	Not available in U.S.
Calcidiol/calcifediol $25(OH)D_3$	Oral	Calderol® Organon Inc.	350-700 per week	
Calcitriol $1\alpha,25(OH)2D_3$	Oral	Rocaltrol® (Roche Laboratories)	*Weekly Dose[25]: iPTH 300-600 pg/mL: 1.5-4.5 iPTH 600-1,000 pg/mL: 3.0-2.0 iPTH >1,000 pg/mL: 9.0-21.0	Generics available
	Intravenous	Calcijex® (Abbott Laboratories)	*Weekly Dose[25]: iPTH 300-600 pg/mL: 1.5-4.5 iPTH 600-1,000 pg/mL: 3.0-9.0 iPTH >1,000 pg/mL: 9.0-15.0	
Cholecalciferol/ Ergocalciferol Vitamin D3/Vitamin D2)	Oral		If 25(OH)D levels <15 ng/mL (37 mmol/L) give 50,000IU weekly for 4 doses and then monthly for 4 doses. If 25(OH)D levels are 15-30 ng/mL give 50,000 IU monthly X 6[25].	Vitamin D_2 may induce less calcium absorption than Vitamin D_3
Dihydrotachysterol (DHT) 25-hydroxydihydrotachysterol	Oral	Hytakerol® Sanofi Synthelabo Inc	Usually in the range of 2 to 14 capsules (0.25 to 1.75 mg) each week	
Doxercalciferol $1\alpha(OH)D_2$	Oral	Hectorol® Capsules Bone Care International	*Weekly Dose[25]: iPTH 300-600 pg/mL: 15.0 iPTH 600-1000 pg/mL: 15.0-30.0 iPTH >1000 pg/mL: 30.0-60.0	Available in U.S. and Canada Only
	Intravenous	Hectorol® Injection Bone Care International	*Weekly Dose[25]: iPTH 300-600 pg/mL: 6.0 iPTH 600-1,000 pg/mL: 6.0-12.0 iPTH >1,000 pg/mL: 12.0-24.0	
Falecalcitriol $1,25(OH)^2 26,27F6\ D_3$	Oral	Fulstan® Tablets Hornel® Tablets	NA	Not available in U.S.
Oxacalcitriol $22\text{-}oxa\text{-}1\alpha,25(OH)_2D_3$	Oral	Maxacalcitol Chugai Pharmaceuticals	15-30 per week[75]	Not available in U.S.
Paricalcitol $1\alpha,25(OH)_2\ 19\text{-}nor\text{-}D_2$	Intravenous	Zemplar® Abbott Laboratories	*Weekly Dose[25]: iPTH 300-600 pg/mL: 7.5-15.0 iPTH 600-1,000 pg/mL: 18.0-30.0 iPTH >1,000 pg/mL: 30.0-45.0	

For intravenous formulation divide weekly dose by 3 for administration at HD. Oral formulations can be administered daily (divide weekly dose by 7) doses or by pulse bolus 3 times per week (divide weekly dose by 3).

Dosage recommendations based on K/DOQI Clinical Practice Guidelines for Bone Metabolism and Disease in CKD. Am J Kidney Dis 42:1-201, 2003.

been extensively studied and its lower calcemic potential might be attributed to VDR selectivity at the tissue level, with higher levels of activity in parathyroid tissue compared to bone or intestine.[57;58] The clinical effectiveness of intravenous paricalcitol has been demonstrated in a controlled clinical trial.[59] A recent uncontrolled, retrospective study, in a large cohort of maintenance hemodialysis patients, showed that paricalcitol conferred a significant survival advantage over calcitriol.[60]

Doxercalciferol

Doxercalciferol (1α-hydroxyvitamin D_2), similar to alfacalcidol, is a prohormone that requires hepatic conversion to its active metabolite, $1,25(OH)_2D_2$. Unlike the supraphysiological blood levels of active D hormone seen with intravenous administration of active D metabolites such as calcitriol and paricalcitol, blood levels of active D metabolites are sustained within the physiologically normal range after administration of doxercalciferol.[61] A pharmacokinetic characteristic of doxercalciferol that might confer a lower calcemic potential is conversion to the active metabolite, $1\alpha24(OH)_2D_2$, which has been shown to have potent prodifferentiation actions and low calcemic potency.[62] The clinical effectiveness of doxercalciferol has been demonstrated with both intravenous and oral administration in hemodialysis, and by oral administration in CKD Stages 3-4. However, the claim of lower calcemic action compared to calcitriol has not been demonstrated definitely.[63-65]

Oxacalcitriol

Oxacalcitriol (22-oxa-$1,25(OH)_2D_3$) is a calcitriol analog developed and commercially available in Japan. In clinical trials, oxacalcitriol effectively reduced intact PTH levels in more than 60% of treated patients without an increase in mean plasma calcium levels.[66] As compared to calcitriol, oxacalcitriol has a lower affinity for the VDR and vitamin D-binding proteins, a shorter plasma half-life, and differences in VDR cofactor requirements. These differences have been taken to indicate lower calcemic activity; however, the claimed lower calcemic action compared to that of calcitriol has not been demonstrated formally.[67]

Falecalcitriol

Falecalcitriol [$1,25(OH)_226,27F\ D_3$] is another vitamin D_3 analog that has the carbons 26 and 27 replaced by fluorine atoms. It is commercially available for oral administration in Japan. In a comparative trial, it had no less calcemic potential than alfacalcidol.[68]

CALCIMIMETICS

Calcimimetics are a promising new class of compounds that act on extracellular calcium-sensing receptors (ECaR) in parathyroid cells, thereby increasing the sensitivity of the gland to extracellular calcium (Figure 1). They lower the threshold for receptor activation by extracellular calcium ions, thereby resulting in suppression of PTH secretion at normal blood calcium levels (Figure 2). In contrast to oral calcium and/or vitamin D therapy, calcimimetics can accomplish this PTH reduction with either no change or even a decrease in plasma calcium and phosphorus levels. A unique characteristic of calcimimetics is that they offer an important new option in treating SHPT without a consequent increase in CaXP.

FIGURE 1. A SCHEMATIC FOR SIGNAL TRANSDUCTION BY EXTRACELLULAR CALCIUM THROUGH THE CaSR

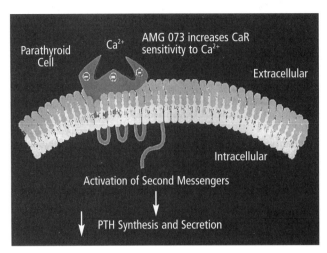

From Goodman WG and Turner SA, Adv. in Renal Replacement Therapy 2002; 9: 200-208. Used with permission.

FIGURE 2. EFFECT OF CALCIMIMETIC AGENTS ON THE PTH-CALCIUM RELATIONSHIP

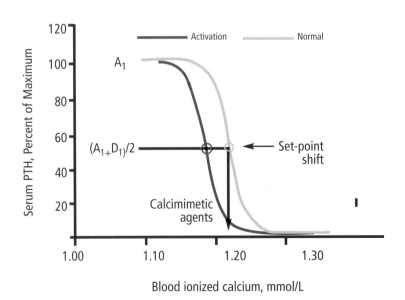

Adapted from Goodman WG, et al. Kidney Int. 1996; 50:1834-1844 (with permission).

Cinacalcet [Sensipar™ (U.S.), Mimpara™ (E.U.)] is the first drug in this class to receive approval for clinical use. Clinical trials have shown that cinacalcet can effectively reduce PTH levels, while simultaneously lowering plasma calcium, phosphorus, and CaXP, in patients on dialysis.[69] The onset of action is rapid with peak reduction in PTH levels occurring 2-6 hours after administration.

Treatment with cinacalcet is generally well tolerated, with nausea and vomiting being the most common side-effects. These can be overcome generally by reducing the initial dose. Hypocalcemia will occur in some patients, and can be managed by adjustments to calcium-based phosphate binders and/or vitamin D sterols.

The recommended starting oral dose of cinacalcet in adults is 30 mg once daily. Plasma calcium and phosphorus should be measured within 1 week and iPTH should be measured 1-4 weeks after initiation or dose adjustment of cinacalcet. The dosage should be titrated no more frequently than every 2-4 weeks, through sequential doses of 60, 90, 120, and 180 mg once daily, to a target iPTH consistent with the NKF-K/DOQI recommendation for CKD patients on dialysis of 150-300 pg/mL (16.5-33 pmol/L). Cinacalcet can be used alone or in combination with vitamin D sterols and/or phosphate binders.[70]

Calcimimetics provide a potentially valuable new treatment option for SHPT, but there is still limited long-term experience and no published evidence of the beneficial effect of this therapy on ROD at the bone level.

PARATHYROIDECTOMY

In the majority of patients, medical management of SHPT will be effective. When medical management is unsuccessful, surgical parathyroidectomy (PTX) can provide effective reduction in PTH. PTX should be considered for patients with severe hyperparathyroidism, defined as persistent elevation of plasma iPTH >800 pg/mL (88.0 pmol/L), associated with hypercalcemia and/or hyperphosphatemia that are refractory to medical therapy.[25] In general, this means patients with severe SHPT who, despite appropriate therapies, have persistent elevations of phosphorus and/or calcium that preclude the use of vitamin D sterols to lower PTH. The recent introduction of calcimimetics offers another valuable treatment alternative for patients for whom PTX is not appropriate. PTX might be considered at lower PTH levels (>500 pg/mL and <800 pg/mL) for patients with significant symptoms such as debilitating pruritus, progressive skeletal and articular pain, and possibly for calciphylaxis[25;71]. In this situation, a bone biopsy may shed additional light on the precise type of associated bone disease and be of value in determining the best course of treatment.

Surgical PTX can be accomplished by subtotal or total PTX, with or without parathyroid tissue auto-transplantation. For parathyroid autotransplantation, the smallest and least nodular gland may be implanted in multiple pockets in muscle, most commonly in the arteriovenous fistula-free forearm.

With the sudden reduction in PTH after PTX, calcium and phosphate influx into bone can increase dramatically, resulting in drops in plasma calcium and phosphorus, a condition referred to as "hungry bone syndrome." The resulting hypocalcemia, which is a frequent complication of the postoperative period, requires close monitoring. In the immediate postoperative period, if ionized or corrected total calcium levels drop below normal (ionized calcium <0.9 mmol/L [3.6 mg/dL] or corrected total calcium <7.2 mg/dL), a calcium gluconate infusion should be initiated at a rate of 1-2 mg elemental calcium per kilogram body weight per hour and adjusted to maintain an ionized calcium in the normal range (1.15-1.36 mmol/L or 4.6-5.4 mg/dL).[25]Alternatively, normal calcium levels can be maintained with oral calcium carbonate 1-2 g TID, as well as oral calcitriol up to 2 μg/day. [25]

Hypophosphatemia is also common after PTX and can usually be managed by discontinuing or reducing any phosphate binders that the patient was receiving preoperatively. Occasionally, severe hypophosphatemia (<1.5-2 mg/dL [0.48-0.64 mmol/L]) occurs and may require phosphate supplementation, keeping in mind that phosphate salts can exacerbate hypocalcemia.[71] PTH plays a role in potassium and magnesium homeostasis; therefore, both hypomagnesemia and hyperkalemia are potential complications following PTX, requiring monitoring and treatment consideration.[71]

Whether due to residual parathyroid tissue or hyperplasia of transplanted tissue, up to one-third of patients will have recurrent SHPT after PTX[72]; thus, ongoing monitoring of bone and mineral metabolism is required.

TREATMENT OPTIONS IN PRESENCE OF ADYNAMIC BONE DISEASE

In addition to having an increased risk of fracture,[2] patients with adynamic bone disease are more prone to acute hypercalcemia and arterial and soft-tissue calcifications.[73;74] Therefore, CKD Stage 5 patients with adynamic bone disease, as documented by bone biopsy or iPTH levels <100 pg/mL (11.0 pmol/L), should be treated by allowing a rise in plasma iPTH levels to increase the rate of bone turnover.[25] This may be accomplished by decreasing/discontinuing vitamin D therapy and/or reducing calcium load. The calcium load can be decreased by reducing or eliminating calcium-based phosphate binders, and, if needed, by lowering the calcium dialysate concentration.

CONCLUSIONS

In the past decade we have seen significant advances in our understanding of the pathophysiology of renal osteodystrophy and associated abnormalities in mineral metabolism. Recent epidemiologic studies have demonstrated the independent relative cardiovascular risk associated with elevations in plasma calcium, PTH and most notably phosphorus. Despite this the current medical management of secondary hyperparathyroidism and hyperphosphatemia remains less than optimal.

The recent introduction of novel drugs, including active vitamin D analogues, non-calcium, non-aluminum based phosphate binders and calcimimetics, should lead to improved clinical management of ROD. In addition to pharmaceutical interventions, it is critical to integrate all available therapeutic options to minimize the complications of ROD. The treatment plan for bone and mineral abnormalities should also include vigorous dietary counseling, optimizing the efficiency of renal replacement therapy and promoting physical exercise.

REFERENCES

1. Block GA, Port FK: Re-evaluation of risks associated with hyperphosphatemia and hyper-parathyroidism in dialysis patients: recommendations for a change in management. Am J Kidney Dis 35:1226-1237, 2000

2. Coco M, Rush H: Increased incidence of hip fractures in dialysis patients with low serum parathyroid hormone. Am J Kidney Dis 36:1115-1121, 2000

3. Malluche HH, Mawad H, Monier-Faugere MC: The importance of bone health in end-stage renal disease: out of the frying pan, into the fire? Nephrol Dial Transplant 19 Suppl 1:i9-13, 2004

4. Mucsi I, Hercz G: Relative hypoparathyroidism and adynamic bone disease. Am J Med Sci 317:405-409, 1999

5. Al Hejaili F, Kortas C, Leitch R, Heidenheim AP, Clement L, Nesrallah G, Lindsay RM: Nocturnal but not short hours quotidian hemodialysis requires an elevated dialysate calcium concentration. J Am Soc Nephrol 14:2322-2328, 2003

6. Llach F, Massry SG: On the mechanism of secondary hyperparathyroidism in moderate renal insufficiency. J Clin Endocrinol Metab 61:601-606, 1985

*7. Slatopolsky E, Brown A, Dusso A: Pathogenesis of secondary hyperparathyroidism. Kidney Int Suppl 73:S14-S19, 1999

8. Wilson L, Felsenfeld A, Drezner MK, Llach F: Altered divalent ion metabolism in early renal failure: role of 1,25(OH)2D. Kidney Int 27:565-573, 1985

9. K/DOQI clinical practice guidelines for chronic kidney disease: evaluation, classification, and stratification. Am J Kidney Dis 39:S1-266, 2002

*10. Hamdy NA, Kanis JA, Beneton MN, Brown CB, Juttmann JR, Jordans JG, Josse S, Meyrier A, Lins RL, Fairey IT: Effect of alfacalcidol on natural course of renal bone disease in mild to moderate renal failure. BMJ 310:358-363, 1995

11. Hutchison AJ, Whitehouse RW, Boulton HF, Adams JE, Mawer EB, Freemont TJ, Gokal R: Correlation of bone histology with parathyroid hormone, vitamin D3, and radiology in end-stage renal disease. Kidney Int 44:1071-1077, 1993

*12. Sherrard DJ, Hercz G, Pei Y, Maloney NA, Greenwood C, Manuel A, Saiphoo C, Fenton SS, Segre GV: The spectrum of bone disease in end-stage renal failure—an evolving disorder. Kidney Int 43:436-442, 1993

13. Atsumi K, Kushida K, Yamazaki K, Shimizu S, Ohmura A, Inoue T: Risk factors for vertebral fractures in renal osteodystrophy. Am J Kidney Dis 33:287-293, 1999

14. Coco M, Rush H: Increased incidence of hip fractures in dialysis patients with low serum parathyroid hormone [In Process Citation]. Am J Kidney Dis 36:1115-1121, 2000

15. Kurz P, Monier-Faugere MC, Bognar B, Werner E, Roth P, Vlachojannis J, Malluche HH: Evidence for abnormal calcium homeostasis in patients with adynamic bone disease. Kidney Int 46:855-861, 1994

16. Blacher J, Demuth K, Guerin AP, Safar ME, Moatti N, London GM: Influence of biochemical alterations on arterial stiffness in patients with end-stage renal disease. Arterioscler Thromb Vasc Biol 18:535-541, 1998

*17. Block GA: Control of serum phosphorus: implications for coronary artery calcification and calcific uremic arteriolopathy (calciphylaxis). Curr Opin Nephrol Hypertens 10:741-747, 2001

18. Goodman WG, Goldin J, Kuizon BD, Yoon C, Gales B, Sider D, Wang Y, Chung J, Emerick A, Greaser L, Elashoff RM, Salusky IB: Coronary-artery calcification in young adults with end-stage renal disease who are undergoing dialysis. N Engl J Med 342:1478-1483, 2000

19. Guerin AP, London GM, Marchais SJ, Metivier F: Arterial stiffening and vascular calcifications in end-stage renal disease. Nephrol Dial Transplant 15:1014-1021, 2000

20. Gutzwiller JP, Schneditz D, Huber AR, Schindler C, Gutzwiller F, Zehnder CE: Estimating phosphate removal in haemodialysis: an additional tool to quantify dialysis dose. Nephrol Dial Transplant 17:1037-1044, 2002

21. Chauveau P, Poignet JL, Kuno T, Bonete R, Kerembrun A, Naret C, Delons S, Man NK, Rist E: Phosphate removal rate: a comparative study of five high-flux dialysers. Nephrol Dial Transplant 6 Suppl 2:114-115, 1991

22. Hou SH, Zhao J, Ellman CF, Hu J, Griffin Z, Spiegel DM, Bourdeau JE: Calcium and phosphorus fluxes during hemodialysis with low calcium dialysate. Am J Kidney Dis 18:217-224, 1991

23. Man NK, Chauveau P, Kuno T, Poignet JL, Yanai M: Phosphate removal during hemodialysis, hemodiafiltration, and hemofiltration. A reappraisal. ASAIO Trans 37:M463-M465, 1991

*24. Mucsi I, Hercz G, Uldall R, Ouwendyk M, Francoeur R, Pierratos A: Control of serum phosphate without any phosphate binders in patients treated with nocturnal hemodialysis. Kidney Int 53:1399-1404, 1998

*25. National Kidney Foundation: K/DOQI clinical practice guidelines for bone metabolism and disease in chronic kidney disease. Am J Kidney Dis 42:1-201, 2003

26. Haag-Weber M: Treatment options to intensify hemodialysis. Kidney Blood Press Res 26:90-95, 2003

27. Lugon JR, Andre MB, Duarte ME, Rembold SM, Cruz E: Effects of in-center daily hemodialysis upon mineral metabolism and bone disease in end-stage renal disease patients. Sao Paulo Med J 119:105-109, 2001

28. Cupisti A, Morelli E, D'Alessandro C, Lupetti S, Barsotti G: Phosphate control in chronic uremia: don't forget diet. J Nephrol 16:29-33, 2003

29. Delmez JA, Slatopolsky E: Hyperphosphatemia: its consequences and treatment in patients with chronic renal disease. Am J Kidney Dis 19:303-317, 1992

30. Wiggins K, American Dietetic Association Renal Practice Group: Guidelines for Nutrition Care of Renal Patients (ed 3rd). Amercian Dietetic Assn, 2001, pp 1-137

*31. Block GA, Klassen PS, Lazarus JM, Ofsthun N, Lowrie EG, Chertow GM: Mineral metabolism, mortality, and morbidity in maintenance hemodialysis. J Am Soc Nephrol 15:2208-2218, 2004

32. Cannata-Andia JB, Fernandez-Martin JL: The clinical impact of aluminium overload in renal failure. Nephrol Dial Transplant 17 Suppl 2:9-12, 2002

*33. Locatelli F, Cannata-Andia JB, Drueke TB, Horl WH, Fouque D, Heimburger O, Ritz E: Management of disturbances of calcium and phosphate metabolism in chronic renal insufficiency, with emphasis on the control of hyperphosphataemia. Nephrol Dial Transplant 17:723-731, 2002

34. Sperschneider H, Gunther K, Marzoll I, Kirchner E, Stein G: Calcium carbonate (CaCO3): an efficient and safe phosphate binder in haemodialysis patients? A 3-year study. Nephrol Dial Transplant 8:530-534, 1993

35. Chertow GM, Burke SK, Lazarus JM, Stenzel KH, Wombolt D, Goldberg D, Bonventre JV, Slatopolsky E: Poly[allylamine hydrochloride] (RenaGel): a noncalcemic phosphate binder for the treatment of hyperphosphatemia in chronic renal failure. Am J Kidney Dis 29:66-71, 1997

36. Slatopolsky EA, Burke SK, Dillon MA: RenaGel, a nonabsorbed calcium- and aluminum-free phosphate binder, lowers serum phosphorus and parathyroid hormone. The RenaGel Study Group. Kidney Int 55:299-307, 1999

37. Burke SK, Dillon MA, Hemken DE, Rezabek MS, Balwit JM: Meta-analysis of the effect of sevelamer on phosphorus, calcium, PTH, and serum lipids in dialysis patients. Adv Ren Replace Ther 10:133-145, 2003

*38. Chertow GM, Burke SK, Raggi P: Sevelamer attenuates the progression of coronary and aortic calcification in hemodialysis patients. Kidney Int 62:245-252, 2002

39. Gallieni M, Cozzolino M, Brancaccio D: Transient decrease of serum bicarbonate levels with Sevelamer hydrochloride as the phosphate binder. Kidney Int 57:1776-1777, 2000

40. Marco MP, Muray S, Betriu A, Craver L, Belart M, Fernandez E: Treatment with sevelamer decreases bicarbonate levels in hemodialysis patients. Nephron 92:499-500, 2002

41. D'Haese PC, Spasovski GB, Sikole A, Hutchison A, Freemont TJ, Sulkova S, Swanepoel C, Pejanovic S, Djukanovic L, Balducci A, Coen G, Sulowicz W, Ferreira A, Torres A, Curic S, Popovic M, Dimkovic N, De Broe ME: A multicenter study on the effects of lanthanum carbonate (Fosrenol) and calcium carbonate on renal bone disease in dialysis patients. Kidney Int Suppl S73-S78, 2003

*42. Joy MS, Finn WF: Randomized, double-blind, placebo-controlled, dose-titration, phase III study assessing the efficacy and tolerability of lanthanum carbonate: a new phosphate binder for the treatment of hyperphosphatemia. Am J Kidney Dis 42:96-107, 2003

43. Lacour B, Lucas A, Auchere D, Ruellan N, Serre Patey NM, Drueke TB: Chronic renal failure is associated with increased tissue deposition of lanthanum after 28-day oral administration. Kidney Int 67:1062-1069, 2005

44. Mai ML, Emmett M, Sheikh MS, Santa Ana CA, Schiller L, Fordtran JS: Calcium acetate, an effective phosphorus binder in patients with renal failure. Kidney Int 36:690-695, 1989

45. Jones G, Strugnell SA, DeLuca HF: Current understanding of the molecular actions of vitamin D. Physiol Rev 78:1193-1231, 1998

46. Przedlacki J, Manelius J, Huttunen K: Bone mineral density evaluated by dual-energy X-ray absorptiometry after one-year treatment with calcitriol started in the predialysis phase of chronic renal failure. Nephron 69:433-437, 1995

*47. Rix M, Eskildsen P, Olgaard K: Effect of 18 months of treatment with alfacalcidol on bone in patients with mild to moderate chronic renal failure. Nephrol Dial Transplant 19:870-876, 2004

*48. Salusky IB, Goodman WG: Adynamic renal osteodystrophy: is there a problem? J Am Soc Nephrol 12:1978-1985, 2001

49. Ishimura E, Nishizawa Y, Inaba M, Matsumoto N, Emoto M, Kawagishi T, Shoji S, Okuno S, Kim M, Miki T, Morii H: Serum levels of 1,25-dihydroxyvitamin D, 24,25-dihydroxyvitamin D, and 25-hydroxyvitamin D in nondialyzed patients with chronic renal failure. Kidney Int 55:1019-1027, 1999

50. Reichel H, Deibert B, Schmidt-Gayk H, Ritz E: Calcium metabolism in early chronic renal failure: implications for the pathogenesis of hyperparathyroidism. Nephrol Dial Transplant 6:162-169, 1991

51. Mazess RB, Elangovan L: A review of intravenous versus oral vitamin D hormone therapy in hemodialysis patients. Clin Nephrol 59:319-325, 2003

52. Quarles LD, Indridason OS: Calcitriol administration in end-stage renal disease: intravenous or oral? Pediatr Nephrol 10:331-336, 1996

53. Brandi L, Daugaard H, Tvedegaard E, Storm T, Olgaard K: Effect of intravenous 1-alpha-hydroxyvitamin D3 on secondary hyperparathyroidism in chronic uremic patients on maintenance hemodialysis. Nephron 53:194-200, 1989

54. Rapoport J, Mostoslavski M, Ben David A, Knecht A, Blau A, Arad J, Zlotnik M, Chaimovitz C: Successful treatment of secondary hyperparathyroidism in hemodialysis patients with oral pulse 1-alpha-hydroxy-cholecalciferol therapy. Nephron 72:150-154, 1996

55. Chan JC, McEnery PT, Chinchilli VM, Abitbol CL, Boineau FG, Friedman AL, Lum GM, Roy S, III, Ruley EJ, Strife CF: A prospective, double-blind study of growth failure in children with chronic renal insufficiency and the effectiveness of treatment with calcitriol versus dihydrotachysterol. The Growth Failure in Children with Renal Diseases Investigators. J Pediatr 124:520-528, 1994

*56. Morii H, Ishimura E, Inoue T, Tabata T, Morita A, Nishii Y, Fukushima M: History of vitamin D treatment of renal osteodystrophy. Am J Nephrol 17:382-386, 1997

57. Finch JL, Brown AJ, Slatopolsky E: Differential effects of 1,25-dihydroxy-vitamin D3 and 19-nor-1,25-dihydroxy-vitamin D2 on calcium and phosphorus resorption in bone. J Am Soc Nephrol 10:980-985, 1999

58. Takahashi F, Finch JL, Denda M, Dusso AS, Brown AJ, Slatopolsky E: A new analog of 1,25-(OH)2D3, 19-NOR-1,25-(OH)2D2, suppresses serum PTH and parathyroid gland growth in uremic rats without elevation of intestinal vitamin D receptor content. Am J Kidney Dis 30:105-112, 1997

59. Martin KJ, Gonzalez EA, Gellens M, Hamm LL, Abboud H, Lindberg J: 19-Nor-1-alpha-25-dihydroxyvitamin D2 (Paricalcitol) safely and effectively reduces the levels of intact parathyroid hormone in patients on hemodialysis. J Am Soc Nephrol 9:1427-1432, 1998

*60. Teng M, Wolf M, Lowrie E, Ofsthun N, Lazarus JM, Thadhani R: Survival of patients under-going hemodialysis with paricalcitol or calcitriol therapy. N Engl J Med 349:446-456, 2003

61. Bailie GR, Johnson CA: Comparative review of the pharmacokinetics of vitamin D ana-logues. Semin Dial 15:352-357, 2002

62. Mawer EB, Jones G, Davies M, Still PE, Byford V, Schroeder NJ, Makin HL, Bishop CW, Knutson JC: Unique 24-hydroxylated metabolites represent a significant pathway of metabolism of vitamin D2 in humans: 24-hydroxyvitamin D2 and 1,24-dihydroxyvitamin D2 detectable in human serum. J Clin Endocrinol Metab 83:2156-2166, 1998

*63. Coburn JW, Maung HM, Elangovan L, Germain MJ, Lindberg JS, Sprague SM, Williams ME, Bishop CW: Doxercalciferol safely suppresses PTH levels in patients with secondary hyperparathyroidism associated with chronic kidney disease stages 3 and 4. Am J Kidney Dis 43:877-890, 2004

64. Frazao JM, Elangovan L, Maung HM, Chesney RW, Acchiardo SR, Bower JD, Kelley BJ, Rodriguez HJ, Norris KC, Robertson JA, Levine BS, Goodman WG, Gentile D, Mazess RB, Kyllo DM, Douglass LL, Bishop CW, Coburn JW: Intermittent doxercalciferol (1alpha-hydroxyvitamin D(2)) therapy for secondary hyperparathyroidism. Am J Kidney Dis 36:550-561, 2000

65. Maung HM, Elangovan L, Frazao JM, Bower JD, Kelley BJ, Acchiardo SR, Rodriguez HJ, Norris KC, Sigala JF, Rutkowski M, Robertson JA, Goodman WG, Levine BS, Chesney RW, Mazess RB, Kyllo DM, Douglass LL, Bishop CW, Coburn JW: Efficacy and side effects of intermittent intravenous and oral doxercalciferol (1alpha-hydroxyvitamin D(2)) in dialysis patients with secondary hyperparathyroidism: a sequential comparison. Am J Kidney Dis 37:532-543, 2001

66. Akizawa T, Suzuki M, Akiba T, Nishizawa Y, Kurokawa K: Clinical effects of maxacalcitol on secondary hyperparathyroidism of uremic patients. Am J Kidney Dis 38:S147-S151, 2001

67. Takeyama K, Masuhiro Y, Fuse H, Endoh H, Murayama A, Kitanaka S, Suzawa M, Yanagisawa J, Kato S: Selective interaction of vitamin D receptor with transcriptional coac-tivators by a vitamin D analog. Mol Cell Biol 19:1049-1055, 1999

68. Akiba T, Marumo F, Owada A, Kurihara S, Inoue A, Chida Y, Ando R, Shinoda T, Ishida Y, Ohashi Y: Controlled trial of falecalcitriol versus alfacalcidol in suppression of parathyroid hormone in hemodialysis patients with secondary hyperparathyroidism. Am J Kidney Dis 32:238-246, 1998

*69. Block GA, Martin KJ, de Francisco AL, Turner SA, Avram MM, Suranyi MG, Hercz G, Cunningham J, Abu-Alfa AK, Messa P, Coyne DW, Locatelli F, Cohen RM, Evenepoel P, Moe SM, Fournier A, Braun J, McCary LC, Zani VJ, Olson KA, Drueke TB, Goodman WG: Cinacalcet for secondary hyperparathyroidism in patients receiving hemodialysis. N Engl J Med 350:1516-1525, 2004

70. Sensipar™ Prescribing Information. Amgen, Thousand Oaks, CA . 2004.
   Ref Type: Abstract

71. Llach F, Bover J: Renal Osteodystophies, in Brenner BM (ed): The Kidney, chap
   51. 2000, pp 2103-2186

*72. Gagne ER, Urena P, Leite-Silva S, Zingraff J, Chevalier A, Sarfati E, Dubost C,
   Drueke TB: Short- and long-term efficacy of total parathyroidectomy with
   immediate autografting compared with subtotal parathyroidectomy in
   hemodialysis patients. J Am Soc Nephrol 3:1008-1017, 1992

*73. London GM, Marty C, Marchais SJ, Guerin AP, Metivier F, de Vernejoul MC:
   Arterial calcifications and bone histomorphometry in end-stage renal disease.
   J Am Soc Nephrol 15:1943-1951, 2004

74. Mawad HW, Sawaya BP, Sarin R, Malluche HH: Calcific uremic arteriolopathy in
   association with low turnover uremic bone disease. Clin Nephrol 52:160-166,
   1999

*75. Hayashi M, Tsuchiya Y, Itaya Y, Takenaka T, Kobayashi K, Yoshizawa M,
   Nakamura R, Monkawa T, Ichihara A: Comparison of the effects of calcitriol
   and maxacalcitol on secondary hyperparathyroidism in patients on chronic
   haemodialysis: a randomized prospective multicentre trial. Nephrol Dial
   Transplant 19:2067-2073, 2004

*Suggested Reading

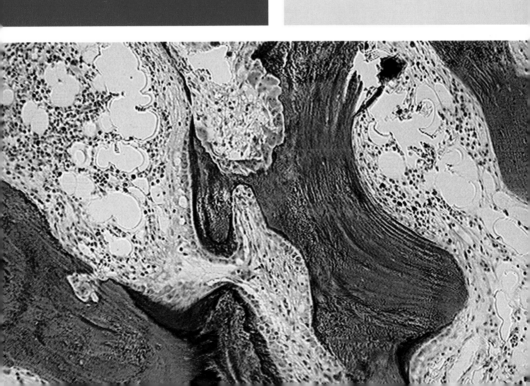

POST-TRANSPLANT
BONE DISEASE

7

Klaus Olgaard
Stuart M. Sprague

CHAPTER 7

POST-TRANSPLANT BONE DISEASE

Klaus Olgaard and Stuart M. Sprague

Disorders of bone and mineral metabolism continue to be a significant clinical problem following kidney transplantation. The majority of transplant recipients have pre-existing disturbances in bone and mineral metabolism secondary to kidney failure and/or diabetes mellitus. These existing disorders are then compounded by the pathological processes that are unique to the post-transplant period (Table 1). Nearly all transplant patients have histological evidence of osteopenia, reduced bone mineral density (BMD), and very high rates of fracture.

TABLE 1. PRE- AND POST-TRANSPLANT RISK FACTORS FOR BONE DISEASE

Pre-transplant risk factors

1. Previous history of renal osteodystrophy:
   a. SHPT
   b. Osteomalacia-hypovitaminosis D
   c. Mixed bone disease
   d. Adynamic bone disease
   e. Aluminum toxicity
2. Drug treatment:
   a. Oversuppression of PTH with active vitamin D analogs and calcium
   b. Previous steroid treatment
   c. Immunosuppressive drugs
   d. Anticonvulsant therapy
3. Other factors:
   a. Immobilization
   b. Malnutrition
   c. Impaired gonadal status
   d. History of fractures
   e. History of musculoskeletal symptoms

Post-transplant risk factors

1. Low GFR post-transplant
2. Immunosuppressive therapy:
   a. Glucocorticoids
   b. Cyclosporin/tacrolimus
3. Persistent hyperparathyroidism
4. Hypercalcemia and hyperphosphatemia
5. Hypophosphatemia/hypomagnesemia
6. Loop diuretics
7. Persistent hypogonadism

Abbreviations: BMD, bone mineral density; DM, diabetes mellitus; GFR, glomerular filtration rate; PTH, parathyroid hormone.

PATHOGENESIS OF BONE DISEASE

There are multiple pathogenic mechanisms for bone disease in the post-transplant period. Nearly all patients will come to transplantation with some degree of bone disease, such as renal osteodystrophy (ROD), which includes secondary hyperparathyroidism (SHPT), adynamic bone disease, aluminum-induced osteomalacia, and amyloidosis. In addition, patients may present with osteoporosis, diabetic osteopathy, and/or abnormalities related to hypogonadism and chronic metabolic acidosis. These underlying bone abnormalities are then compounded by post-transplant immunosuppressive therapy, disorders of mineral metabolism, continued poor kidney function, and ongoing hyperparathyroidism.

Immunosuppressive Therapy

The rapid loss of bone mass following transplant has been primarily attributed to glucocorticoid and other immunosuppressive therapies. BMD declines by as much as 10% after transplantation, with most of the loss occurring in the first 6-12 months. The degree of bone loss is directly related to the dose and duration of glucocorticoid exposure. Long-term glucocorticoid administration directly inhibits bone formation by decreasing osteoblast recruitment and differentiation, inducing apoptosis in mature osteoblasts, and inhibiting the synthesis of Type I collagen. Glucocorticoids can directly enhance osteoclastic activity as well, resulting in increased bone resorption.[1,2] While this direct effect on resorption is not as pronounced as the suppression of bone formation, glucocorticoids also indirectly stimulate bone resorption by means of their inhibition of gonadal steroids. Glucocorticoids reduce plasma calcium levels by inhibiting renal 1,25-dihydroxycholecalciferol (calcitriol) synthesis, decreasing intestinal calcium absorption, and increasing urinary calcium excretion, which results in a negative calcium balance, increased parathyroid hormone (PTH) secretion, and greater bone resorption.

The effects of other immunosuppressive therapies on bone are not as clearly established. The calcineurin inhibitors, cyclosporine (CsA), and tacrolimus (FK-506) suppress T-cell function and are effective in reducing post-transplant rejection episodes. CsA may contribute to post-transplant bone loss, as it has been associated with high turnover osteopenia in rat models[3]; however, in in vitro models it appears to inhibit bone resorption,[4] and clinical studies in transplant recipients have not uniformly supported bone loss in humans.[5-7] Tacrolimus has shown similar bone loss properties in rats.[8] The effect of tacrolimus on the human skeleton following kidney transplantion is not well studied, but it may cause less bone loss compared to immunosuppressive regimens with CsA.[9-12]

The effects of other immunosuppressive drugs—sirolimus (rapamycin), mycophenolate mofetil, and azathioprine—on bone metabolism have not been as thoroughly evaluated. They appear to have little or no effect on bone mass.[5,13-16]

Mineral Imbalances

Hypophosphatemia is a frequent problem following kidney transplantion.[17] It is primarily due to dysregulation of sodium-dependent phosphate transport in the proximal tubule, resulting in hyperphosphaturia. Elevated PTH levels, low calcitriol levels, and glucocorticoid therapy can all contribute to this excessive urinary phosphorus excretion, and high levels of a newly identified hormonal regulator, phosphatonin, may also play an important role and contribute to post–renal transplant hypophosphatemia.[18] This regulator has been recently recognized to be FGF-23. In renal transplant recipients, its circulating concentration increases with declining renal function, as it does in CKD patients who have not received transplants.[19] In addition to exacerbating osteopenia and osteomalacia, persistent hypophosphatemia can lead to cardiac arrhythmias and impaired contractility, respiratory failure, and neurological complications.[20]

Hypercalcemia is also common following kidney transplantion, primarily due to persistence of pre-existing hyperparathyroidism. Additional factors that may contribute to hypercalcemia include the effect of high-dose glucocorticoids, postoperative immobility, hypophosphatemia, and resolution of soft-tissue calcifications.[21;22] With return of kidney function, there is an increased sensitivity to the calcemic action of PTH, resulting in increased calcium resorption from bone, enhanced calcium reabsorption in the kidney, and an indirect increase in intestinal calcium absorption due to increased calcitriol production. The hypercalcemia will usually resolve as the parathyroid gland function normalizes; however, in a small number of patients, hypercalcemia may persist.

Metabolic Acidosis

There are a variety of causes for persistent metabolic acidosis following kidney transplantation, such as renal tubular acidosis, persistent uremia, diabetic ketoacidosis due to post-transplant diabetes mellitus, and acidosis due to ischemia or nephrotoxicity. The skeletal buffering mechanism compensates for the acidosis, leading to further depletion of bone mineral content and altered bone remodeling. Correction of post-transplant acidosis is important to minimize this component of bone loss.

Kidney Function

Another very important consideration in the evolution of post-transplant bone disease is the glomerular filtration rate (GFR). Patients who do not achieve a GFR >70 mL/min/1.73 m^2 are at greater risk for persistent hyperparathyroidism and progression of ROD.[23;24] Even in those who achieve a GFR >70 mL/min/1.73 m^2, the subsequent loss of kidney function due to chronic allograph nephropathy results in the onset of ROD due to the progressive loss of kidney function.

Hyperparathyroidism

With a functioning renal allograft, hyperphosphatemia generally resolves and production of calcitriol resumes, with beneficial effects on SHPT. Experimentally, normalization of the parathyroid function takes place after a successful kidney transplantation,[25] and the majority of patients will experience a rapid initial decline in PTH levels and full normalization within a year after transplant. However, elevated PTH levels persist in a large number of renal transplant patients or recur in those who lose kidney function due to chronic rejection. In addition to its potential negative consequences on bone mineralization, persistent hyperparathyroidism can worsen hypercalcemia, hypophosphatemia, and may be a risk factor for acute tubular necrosis in renal allografts.[26] Approximately 5% of kidney transplant patients require an intervention to reduce PTH levels, e.g., a parathyroidectomy, or (in the future) treatment with calcimimetics.[27] General criteria for a post-transplant parathyroidectomy are symptomatic hypercalcemia or asymptomatic hypercalcemia with persistent elevation of PTH levels 1 year following transplant.[22;28]

MANIFESTATIONS OF BONE DISEASE

Fracture Rates

Patients with chronic kidney disease prior to transplantation are at increased risk of fracture, with a vertebral fracture prevalence as high as 21% and the relative risk of hip fracture increased by 2- to 14-fold.[29;30] Following successful kidney transplantation, studies report fracture rates between 5% and 44%, with a nearly four-fold increase in fracture rates from the pretransplant period (0.009 per patient year) to the post-transplant period (0.032 per patient year).[31;32] Patients with diabetes receiving a kidney graft have post-transplantation fracture rates as high as 40% and 49%.[33;34] Post-transplant duration of time is associated with increasing fracture rates.[35] Post-transplant fractures have a significant impact on patient rehabilitation, morbidity, and health-care costs; therefore, post-transplant medical management must include measures to minimize risk factors.

Bone Mineral Density

Following transplantation, most often BMD decreases dramatically for the first 6 months and then the bone loss tends to slow or even recover in the subsequent 6-18 months.[36;37] Bone loss is variable at different sites and, while more pronounced in trabecular bone (lumbar spine), there is also loss in sites with predominantly cortical bone (femoral neck).[36;38;39] The most significant risk factor for post-transplant bone loss is total glucocorticoid exposure.[6;40]

Light Microscopy Findings

Post-transplant bone biopsies are uncommon in clinical practice, but are the only way to obtain specific information on the pathophysiological mechanism and magnitude of skeletal problems. Although bone mineral loss following transplantation is quite consistent, the bone pathology involved is highly variable, as demonstrated by the heterogeneous findings of bone biopsy studies. Histological findings associated with the rapid loss in bone mass in the first 6 months after transplantation include a marked decrease in mineral apposition and bone formation, resulting in prolongation of mineralization lag time and formation periods, with a reduction of elevated pretransplant resorption rates.[37] This pattern is consistent with adynamic bone disease. Studies conducted in patients with long-term transplantation have also shown low-turnover bone disease, with decreased bone formation and prolonged mineralization lag time, but normal resorption activities and evidence of osteomalacia. This pattern suggests defective osteoblast function and/or survival.[41] Many patients also show histological evidence of high-turnover bone disease.[42;43] Biochemical bone markers, while useful, are not consistently reliable in predicting the type of bone disease. Histological findings can provide valuable information to refine treatment decisions in an individual patient.

Avascular Necrosis

Avascular necrosis (AVN) is a serious complication after transplantation. The femoral head is the most common site of occurrence, but other weight-bearing joints can be affected.[44] The pathogenesis for the disruption of blood flow in this ischemic bone disease is not well elucidated. A possible mechanism is the proliferation of fat cells within critical areas of the marrow space, increasing intraosseous pressure, and thereby interfering with bone perfusion.[44] Larger doses of glucocorticoids and longer duration on dialysis prior to transplantation appear to be risk factors for the development of AVN.[45;46] The frequency of post-transplant AVN has been declining in recent years to approximately 5%, likely due to more cautious glucocorticoid dosing.[47]

PROPHYLAXIS AND TREATMENT OF POST-TRANSPLANT BONE DISEASE

Since the most rapid bone loss occurs immediately after transplantation, it is important to institute preventive measures as soon as possible. Table 1 provides an overview of pre- and post-transplant risk factors that should be considered when determining a treatment plan for bone and mineral disorders following transplant. There are no established therapies and few clinical studies on which to base treatment of bone disease following kidney transplant. Treatment recommendations are therefore primarily opinion-based; they are derived from clinical experience, and extrapolation from clinical study data obtained by therapeutic interventions in the general population and in patients with other solid organ transplantations (Table 2).

TABLE 2. TREATMENT/PROPHYLAXIS FOR POST-TRANSPLANT BONE DISEASE

1. General
   a. Tailor immunosuppressive therapy
      i. Use the lowest possible steroids dose and consider alternate-day therapy
      ii. Use "bone-sparing steroids"
   b. Avoid loop diuretics, if possible
      i. Use thiazides
   c. Restore gonadal/thyroid function
   d. Stop smoking
   e. Initiate exercise
   f. Treat persistent hyperparathyroidism
      i. Optimal management of calcium
      ii. Optimal management of vitamin D
      iii. Possible role of calcimimetics
      iv. Parathyroidectomy
   g. Treat other causes of hypercalcemia
   h. Treat persistent hypophosphatemia
   i. Treat persistent hypomagnesemia
2. Vitamin D
   a. Cholecalciferol or ergocalciferol 600 to 1,200 units per day
   b. Active vitamin D compounds
      i. Alfacalcidol
      ii. Calcitriol
      iii. Doxercalciferol
      iv. Paricalcitol
3. Calcium supplementation
   a. Calcium intake of 1,000 mg per day
   b. Post-menopausal women 1,500 mg per day
4. Bisphosphonates
   a. Use of bisphosphonates might be considered:
      i. As treatment of severe osteopenia or fractures in patients with a stable GFR >50-60 mL/min/1.73 m^2
      ii. As would be the treatment for severe postmenopausal osteoporosis?
      iii. As prophylaxis, although data is sparse
   b. Bisphosphonates should be avoided
      i. When GFR is <40 mL/min/m^2
      ii. In the presence of secondary or tertiary HPT
      iii. In the presence of hypovitaminosis D
      iv. In premenopausal women

Abbreviations: GFR, glomerular filtration rate; HPT, hyperparathyroidism.

Calcium

Patients with normal plasma calcium levels should have a daily calcium intake of at least 1,000 mg per day for males and 1,500 mg per day for post-menopausal females. In patients receiving diuretics, thiazide diuretics may be preferable to furosemide due to their calcium-sparing properties.

Vitamin D

In patients with good kidney function and without persistent hypercalcemia, low-dose vitamin D in the form of cholecalciferol or ergocalciferol (600 to 800 units per day) can have prophylactic benefits to minimize glucocorticoid-induced osteopenia. Small doses of active vitamin D derivatives—alfacalcidol, doxercalciferol, or calcitriol (0.25-0.5 µg/daily or every other day)—may also be considered. Alfacalcidol has been shown to prevent bone loss and reduce fracture rates in glucocorticoid-treated patients.[48;49] Calcitriol, used with calcium supplementation, has also been shown to mitigate the bone loss following transplantation in a blinded, double-placebo-controlled study.[11] Vitamin D metabolites may mitigate the bone wasting effect of glucocorticoids by enhancing calcium absorption and reducing PTH secretion.

Bisphosphonates

It is well established that bisphosphonates have beneficial effects in the prevention and treatment of glucocorticoid-induced bone loss.[50;51] Several small studies have suggested the benefit of bisphosphonates in maintaining BMD after kidney transplant, both in the immediate transplant period[36;52] and later in the course of recovery.[53;54] There remains much more to be learned about the most appropriate use of bisphosphonates in kidney transplant patients, including the following parameters: dose, route and timing of administration; contraindications depending on kidney function impairment and type of underlying bone disease; and use in pediatric patients. Use of bisphosphonates might induce adynamic bone disease, and they should probably not be given without a previous bone biopsy.[55] Bisphosphonates should not be used in pre-menopausal women. At this time, it seems reasonable to consider bisphosphonate therapy in other transplant patients with high risk for bone disease, including postmenopausal women with documented severe osteoporosis and patients with pre-existing fractures.

Calcitonin

Calcitonin is a naturally occurring hormone with antiresorptive actions. It has been used to treat conventional osteoporosis, and there have been a few small studies reporting a benefit on post-transplant bone disease.[56;57]

Other Preventive or Therapeutic Considerations

There is no clear evidence to put forward a definitive bone-sparing immunosuppressive regimen, but any regimen that reduces the total exposure to glucocorticoids can potentially reduce post-transplant bone loss. Hypogonadism is common in CKD, and can persist into the post-transplant period. Consideration should be given to estrogen or testosterone replacement therapy in selected cases. Immobilization is very detrimental to bone health, so it is essential to promote exercise and weight-bearing activities in the post-transplant period. Cinacalcet, a type II calcimimetic, is effective in reducing PTH levels in dialysis patients.[27;58] It may also be useful in the post-transplant patient with persistent hyperparathyroidism.[59]

CONCLUSIONS

Post-transplant bone and mineral disorders significantly impact the quality of life of kidney transplant patients. The most rapid bone loss occurs in the first 6 months after transplant, so evaluation and intervention needs to be a part of the immediate postsurgical period. The etiology of bone disease after transplant is complex and multi-factorial, making it difficult to develop a treatment protocol that is simple and widely applicable. There remains much to do in clinical research and much to be learned in this area, as demonstrated by the limited evidence base of the K/DOQI Clinical Practice Guidelines for Bone Metabolism and Disease in CKD with regard to post-transplant bone disease (Table 3),[60] and from the European Best Practice Guidelines for Renal Transplantation (Part 2).[61]

TABLE 3. K/DOQI CLINICAL GUIDELINES FOR POST-TRANPLANT BONE DISEASE[60]

1. Serum levels of calcium, phosphorus, total CO_2 and plasma intact PTH should be monitored following kidney transplantation. (OPINION)

   a. The frequency of these measurements should be based on the time following transplantation, as shown in Table 33. (OPINION)

   Table 33. Frequency of Measurement of Calcium, Phosphorus, PTH, and Total CO_2 after Kidney Transplantation.

Parameter	First 3 Months	3 Months to 1 Year
Calcium	Every 2 weeks	Monthly
Phosphorus	Every 2 weeks	Monthly
PTH	Monthly	Every 3 months
Total CO_2	Every 2 weeks	Monthly

   One year after transplantation, the frequency of measurements should follow the recommendations of Tables 14 and 15, Guideline 1, depending on the level of kidney function.

2. During the first week after kidney transplantation, serum levels of phosphorus should be measured daily. Kidney transplant recipients who develop persistently low levels of serum phosphate (<2.5 mg/dL [0.81 mmol/L]) should be treated with phosphate supplementation. (OPINION)

3. To minimize bone mass loss and **osteonecrosis**, the immunosuppressive regimen should be adjusted to the lowest effective dose of **glucocorticoids**. (EVIDENCE)

4. Kidney transplant recipients should have bone mineral density (BMD) measured by dual energy X-ray **absorptiometry** (DEXA) to assess the presence or development of osteoporosis. (OPINION)

   a. DEXA scans should be obtained at time of transplant, 1 year, and 2 years post-transplant. (OPINION)

   b. If BMD t-score is equal to or less than -2 at the time of the transplant or at subsequent evaluations, therapy with **parenteral** amino-bisphosphonates should be considered. (OPINION)

5. Treatment of disturbances in bone and mineral metabolism is determined by the level of kidney function in the transplant recipient as provided in Guidelines 1 through 15 for CKD patients. (OPINION)

Abbreviations: CKD, chronic kidney disease; PTH, parathyroid hormone.

REFERENCES

1. Canalis E: Clinical review 83: Mechanisms of glucocorticoid action in bone: implications to glucocorticoid-induced osteoporosis. J Clin Endocrinol Metab 81:3441-3447, 1996

2. Moe SM: The treatment of steroid-induced bone loss in transplantation. Curr Opin Nephrol Hypertens 6:544-549, 1997

3. Epstein S: Post-transplantation bone disease: the role of immunosuppressive agents and the skeleton. J Bone Miner Res 11:1-7, 1996

4. Stewart PJ, Stern PH: Cyclosporines: correlation of immunosuppressive activity and inhibition of bone resorption. Calcif Tissue Int 45:222-226, 1989

5. Westeel FP, Mazouz H, Ezaitouni F, Hottelart C, Ivan C, Fardellone P, Brazier M, El E, I, Petit J, Achard JM, Pruna A, Fournier A: Cyclosporine bone remodeling effect prevents steroid osteopenia after kidney transplantation. Kidney Int 58:1788-1796, 2000

6. McIntyre HD, Menzies B, Rigby R, Perry-Keene DA, Hawley CM, Hardie IR: Long-term bone loss after renal transplantation: comparison of immunosuppressive regimens. Clin Transplant 9:20-24, 1995

7. Grotz W, Mundinger A, Gugel B, Exner V, Reichelt A, Schollmeyer P: Missing impact of cyclosporine on osteoporosis in renal transplant recipients. Transplant Proc 26:2652-2653, 1994

8. Cvetkovic M, Mann GN, Romero DF, Liang XG, Ma Y, Jee WS, Epstein S: The deleterious effects of long-term cyclosporine A, cyclosporine G, and FK506 on bone mineral metabolism in vivo. Transplantation 57:1231-1237, 1994

9. Goffin E, Devogelaer JP, Lalaoui A, Depresseux G, De Naeyer P, Squifflet JP, Pirson Y, van Ypersele dS: Tacrolimus and low-dose steroid immunosuppression preserves bone mass after renal transplantation. Transpl Int 15:73-80, 2002

10. Goffin E, Devogelaer JP, Depresseux G, Squifflet JP, Pirson Y, van Yperselede dS: Evaluation of bone mineral density after renal transplantation under a tacrolimus-based immunosuppression: a pilot study. Clin Nephrol 59:190-195, 2003

11. Josephson MA, Schumm LP, Chiu MY, Marshall C, Thistlethwaite JR, Sprague SM: Calcium and calcitriol prophylaxis attenuates posttransplant bone loss. Transplantation 78:1233-1236, 2004

12. Monegal A, Navasa M, Guanabens N, Peris P, Pons F, Martinez de Osaba MJ, Rimola A, Rodes J, Munoz-Gomez J: Bone mass and mineral metabolism in liver transplant patients treated with FK506 or cyclosporine A. Calcif Tissue Int 68:83-86, 2001

13. Aroldi A, Tarantino A, Montagnino G, Cesana B, Cocucci C, Ponticelli C: Effects of three immunosuppressive regimens on vertebral bone density in renal transplant recipients: a prospective study. Transplantation 63:380-386, 1997

14. Bryer HP, Isserow JA, Armstrong EC, Mann GN, Rucinski B, Buchinsky FJ, Romero DF, Epstein S: Azathioprine alone is bone sparing and does not alter cyclosporin A-induced osteopenia in the rat. J Bone Miner Res 10:132-138, 1995

*15. Goodman GR, Dissanayake IR, Sodam BR, Gorodetsky E, Lu J, Ma YF, Jee WS, Epstein S: Immunosuppressant use without bone loss—implications for bone loss after transplantation. J Bone Miner Res 16:72-78, 2001

16. Joffe I, Katz I, Sehgal S, Bex F, Kharode Y, Tamasi J, Epstein S: Lack of change of cancellous bone volume with short-term use of the new immunosuppressant rapamycin in rats. Calcif Tissue Int 53:45-52, 1993

17. Levi M: Post-transplant hypophosphatemia. Kidney Int 59:2377-2387, 2001

18. Green J, Debby H, Lederer E, Levi M, Zajicek HK, Bick T: Evidence for a PTH-independent humoral mechanism in post-transplant hypophosphatemia and phosphaturia. Kidney Int 60:1182-1196, 2001

19. Larsson T, Nisbeth U, Ljunggren O, Juppner H, Jonsson KB: Circulating concentration of FGF-23 increases as renal function declines in patients with chronic kidney disease, but does not change in response to variation in phosphate intake in healthy volunteers. Kidney Int 64:2272-2279, 2003

20. Rubin MF, Narins RG: Hypophosphatemia: pathophysiological and practical aspects of its therapy. Semin Nephrol 10:536-545, 1990

21. McGregor D, Burn J, Lynn K, Robson R: Rapid resolution of tumoral calcinosis after renal transplantation. Clin Nephrol 51:54-58, 1999

22. Parfitt AM: Hypercalcemic hyperparathyroidism following renal transplantation: differential diagnosis, management, and implications for cell population control in the parathyroid gland. Miner Electrolyte Metab 8:92-112, 1982

23. Reinhardt W, Bartelworth H, Jockenhovel F, Schmidt-Gayk H, Witzke O, Wagner K, Heemann UW, Reinwein D, Philipp T, Mann K: Sequential changes of biochemical bone parameters after kidney transplantation. Nephrol Dial Transplant 13:436-442, 1998

24. Rix M, Lewin E, Olgaard K: Posttransplant bone disease. Transplantation Reviews 17:176-186, 2003

25. Lewin E: Involution of the parathyroid glands after renal transplantation. Curr Opin Nephrol Hypertens 12:363-371, 2003

26. Traindl O, Langle F, Reading S, Franz M, Watschinger B, Klauser R, Woloszczuk W, Kovarik J: Secondary hyperparathyroidism and acute tubular necrosis following renal transplantation. Nephrol Dial Transplant 8:173-176, 1993

27. Lindberg JS, Moe SM, Goodman WG, Coburn JW, Sprague SM, Liu W, Blaisdell PW, Brenner RM, Turner SA, Martin KJ: The calcimimetic AMG 073 reduces parathyroid hormone and calcium x phosphorus in secondary hyperparathyroidism. Kidney Int 63:248-254, 2003

28. D'Alessandro AM, Melzer JS, Pirsch JD, Sollinger HW, Kalayoglu M, Vernon WB, Belzer FO, Starling JR: Tertiary hyperparathyroidism after renal transplantation: operative indications. Surgery 106:1049-1055, 1989

29. Alem AM, Sherrard DJ, Gillen DL, Weiss NS, Beresford SA, Heckbert SR, Wong C, Stehman-Breen C: Increased risk of hip fracture among patients with end-stage renal disease. Kidney Int 58:396-399, 2000

30. Stehman-Breen CO, Sherrard DJ, Alem AM, Gillen DL, Heckbert SR, Wong CS, Ball A, Weiss NS: Risk factors for hip fracture among patients with end-stage renal disease. Kidney Int 58:2200-2205, 2000

31. Grotz WH, Mundinger FA, Gugel B, Exner V, Kirste G, Schollmeyer PJ: Bone fracture and osteodensitometry with dual energy X-ray absorptiometry in kidney transplant recipients. Transplantation 58:912-915, 1994

32. Ramsey-Goldman R, Dunn JE, Dunlop DD, Stuart FP, Abecassis MM, Kaufman DB, Langman CB, Salinger MH, Sprague SM: Increased risk of fracture in patients receiving solid organ transplants. J Bone Miner Res 14:456-463, 1999

33. Chiu MY, Sprague SM, Bruce DS, Woodle ES, Thistlethwaite JR, Jr., Josephson MA: Analysis of fracture prevalence in kidney-pancreas allograft recipients. J Am Soc Nephrol 9:677-683, 1998

34. Nisbeth U, Lindh E, Ljunghall S, Backman U, Fellstrom B: Increased fracture rate in diabetes mellitus and females after renal transplantation. Transplantation 67:1218-1222, 1999

*35. Sprague SM, Josephson MA: Bone disease after kidney transplantation. Semin Nephrol 24:82-90, 2004

36. Fan SL, Almond MK, Ball E, Evans K, Cunningham J: Pamidronate therapy as prevention of bone loss following renal transplantation1. Kidney Int 57:684-690, 2000

37. Julian BA, Laskow DA, Dubovsky J, Dubovsky EV, Curtis JJ, Quarles LD: Rapid loss of verte- bral mineral density after renal transplantation. N Engl J Med 325:544-550, 1991

38. Almond MK, Kwan JT, Evans K, Cunningham J: Loss of regional bone mineral density in the first 12 months following renal transplantation. Nephron 66:52-57, 1994

39. Kwan JT, Almond MK, Evans K, Cunningham J: Changes in total body bone mineral content and regional bone mineral density in renal patients following renal transplantation. Miner Electrolyte Metab 18:166-168, 1992

*40. Patel S, Kwan JT, McCloskey E, McGee G, Thomas G, Johnson D, Wills R, Ogunremi L, Barron J: Prevalence and causes of low bone density and fractures in kidney transplant patients. J Bone Miner Res 16:1863-1870, 2001

*41. Bellorin-Font E, Rojas E, Carlini RG, Suniaga O, Weisinger JR: Bone remodeling after renal transplantation. Kidney Int Suppl S125-S128, 2003

*42. Cueto-Manzano AM, Konel S, Hutchison AJ, Crowley V, France MW, Freemont AJ, Adams JE, Mawer B, Gokal R: Bone loss in long-term renal transplantation: histopathology and densitometry analysis. Kidney Int 55:2021-2029, 1999

43. Parker CR, Freemont AJ, Blackwell PJ, Grainge MJ, Hosking DJ: Cross-sectional analysis of renal transplantation osteoporosis. J Bone Miner Res 14:1943-1951, 1999

44. Ficat RP: Idiopathic bone necrosis of the femoral head. Early diagnosis and treatment. J Bone Joint Surg Br 67:3-9, 1985

45. Felson DT, Anderson JJ: Across-study evaluation of association between steroid dose and bolus steroids and avascular necrosis of bone. Lancet 1:902-906, 1987

46. Lauston G, Jensen J, Olgaard K: Necrosis of the femoral head after transplantation. Acta Orthop Scand 59:650-654, 1988

47. Lausten GS, Lemser T, Jensen PK, Egfjord M: Necrosis of the femoral head after kidney transplantation. Clin Transplant 12:572-574, 1998

48. Reginster JY, de Froidmont C, Lecart MP, Sarlet N, Defraigne JO: Alphacalcidol in prevention of glucocorticoid-induced osteoporosis. Calcif Tissue Int 65:328-331, 1999

49. Ringe JD, Coster A, Meng T, Schacht E, Umbach R: Treatment of glucocorticoid-induced osteoporosis with alfacalcidol/calcium versus vitamin D/calcium. Calcif Tissue Int 65:337-340, 1999

50. Roux C, Oriente P, Laan R, Hughes RA, Ittner J, Goemaere S, Di Munno O, Pouilles JM, Horlait S, Cortet B: Randomized trial of effect of cyclical etidronate in the prevention of corticosteroid-induced bone loss. Ciblos Study Group. J Clin Endocrinol Metab 83:1128-1133, 1998

51. Saag KG, Emkey R, Schnitzer TJ, Brown JP, Hawkins F, Goemaere S, Thamsborg G, Liberman UA, Delmas PD, Malice MP, Czachur M, Daifotis AG: Alendronate for the prevention and treatment of glucocorticoid-induced osteoporosis. Glucocorticoid-Induced Osteoporosis Intervention Study Group. N Engl J Med 339:292-299, 1998

52. Haas M, Leko-Mohr Z, Roschger P, Kletzmayr J, Schwarz C, Mitterbauer C, Steininger R, Grampp S, Klaushofer K, Delling G, Oberbauer R: Zoledronic acid to prevent bone loss in the first 6 months after renal transplantation. Kidney Int 63:1130-1136, 2003

53. Arlen DJ, Lambert K, Ioannidis G, Adachi JD: Treatment of established bone loss after renal transplantation with etidronate. Transplantation 71:669-673, 2001

*54. Grotz W, Nagel C, Poeschel D, Cybulla M, Petersen KG, Uhl M, Strey C, Kirste G, Olschewski M, Reichelt A, Rump LC: Effect of ibandronate on bone loss and renal function after kidney transplantation. J Am Soc Nephrol 12:1530-1537, 2001

55. Coco M, Glicklich D, Faugere MC, Burris L, Bognar I, Durkin P, Tellis V, Greenstein S, Schechner R, Figueroa K, McDonough P, Wang G, Malluche H: Prevention of bone loss in renal transplant recipients: a prospective, randomized trial of intravenous pamidronate. J Am Soc Nephrol 14:2669-2676, 2003

56. Grotz WH, Rump LC, Niessen A, Schmidt-Gayk H, Reichelt A, Kirste G, Olschewski M, Schollmeyer PJ: Treatment of osteopenia and osteoporosis after kidney transplantation. Transplantation 66:1004-1008, 1998

57. Ugur A, Guvener N, Isiklar I, Karakayali H, Erdal R: Efficiency of preventive treatment for osteoporosis after renal transplantation. Transplant Proc 32:556-557, 2000

58. Block GA, Martin KJ, de Francisco AL, Turner SA, Avram MM, Suranyi MG, Hercz G, Cunningham J, Abu-Alfa AK, Messa P, Coyne DW, Locatelli F, Cohen RM, Evenepoel P, Moe SM, Fournier A, Braun J, McCary LC, Zani VJ, Olson KA, Drueke TB, Goodman WG: Cinacalcet for secondary hyperparathyroidism in patients receiving hemodialysis. N Engl J Med 350:1516-1525, 2004

59. Kruse AE, Eisenberger U, Frey FJ, Mohaupt MG: The calcimimetic cinacalcet normalizes serum calcium in renal transplant patients with persistent hyperparathyroidism. Nephrol Dial Transplant 20:1311-1314, 2005

60. National Kidney Foundation: K/DOQI clinical practice guidelines for bone metabolism and disease in chronic kidney disease. Am J Kidney Dis 42: 4 Suppl 3:1-201, 2003

61. European best practice guidelines for renal transplantation. Section IV: Long-term management of the transplant recipient. IV.8. Bone disease. Nephrol Dial Transplant 17 Suppl 4:43-48, 2002

*Suggested Reading

RENAL
OSTEODYSTROPHY
IN CHILDREN

Isidro Salusky
Otto Mehls

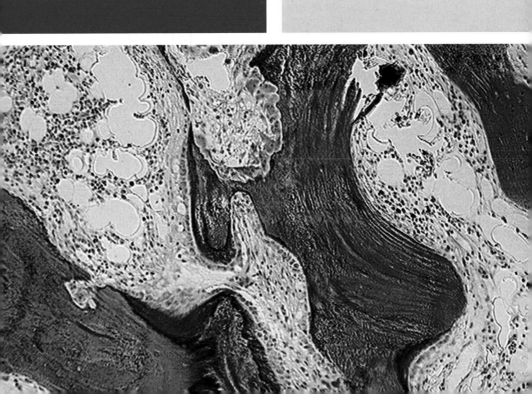

CHAPTER 8

RENAL OSTEODYSTROPHY IN CHILDREN

Isidro Salusky and Otto Mehls

Metabolic bone disease is a significant clinical problem in children with CKD. In an observational study of 247 Dutch patients with onset of CKD before the age of 14 years, more than 60% had severe (greater than -2 SD) growth retardation, 36.8% had clinical symptoms of bone disease, and 17.8% were disabled as a result of their bone disease.[1]

The pathophysiological mechanisms underlying the abnormalities in bone and mineral metabolism that accompany uremia are similar in adults and children. However, there are distinct differences in the clinical manifestations of renal bone disease in children, primarily due to the active growth state of the skeleton. In addition to disturbances in calcium/phosphorus metabolism, production of 1,25-dihyroxyvitamin D (calcitriol), and parathyroid function, progressive uremia affects levels of and sensitivity to hormones that impact both longitudinal bone growth and appositional modeling. Bony deformities and abnormal linear bone growth and growth velocity are significant problems. The spectrum of renal osteodystrophy (ROD) also differs in children, with high-turnover bone disease related to hyperparathyroidism being predominant. Adynamic bone is not as common in children as in adults, though the prevalence is higher in children treated with intermittent, large doses of calcitriol and calcium-based phosphate binders.[2]

The goals of treating bone disease in children with CKD are to attain optimal skeletal growth and control the spectrum of ROD. At the same time, treatment should prevent the development of soft-tissue and vascular calcifications related to disturbances in bone and mineral metabolism.

NORMAL GROWTH AND DEVELOPMENT OF THE SKELETON

During childhood, long bones grow both in length and diameter. Longitudinal growth is dependent on the proliferation of cartilage cells in the epiphyseal growth plates at both the proximal and distal ends of long bones. During growth, there is a continual process along each growth plate where chondrocytes proliferate, mature, hypertrophy, and eventually die (Figure 1). The area around the apoptotic chondrocytes then undergoes a process of matrix formation and mineralization. This endochondral ossification is influenced by multiple hormones and local factors. Ultimately, the balance between proliferation and maturation shifts towards maturation after puberty, and the area of proliferating chondrocytes declines until the

FIGURE 1. GROWTH PLATE

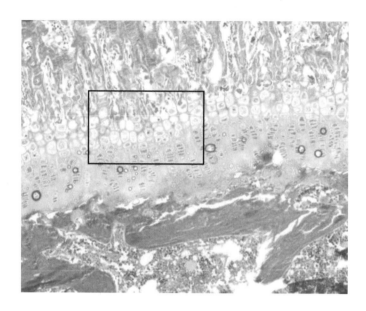

Reproduced with permission from: University of Aberdeen, Histology and EM Core Facility, Online at: http://www.abdn.ac.uk/ims/h-em/images/gallery-figure2.jpg

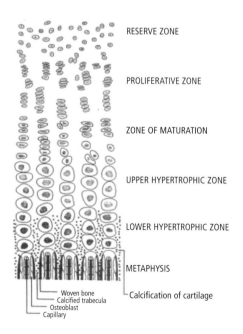

RESERVE ZONE

PROLIFERATIVE ZONE

ZONE OF MATURATION

UPPER HYPERTROPHIC ZONE

LOWER HYPERTROPHIC ZONE

METAPHYSIS

Calcification of cartilage

Woven bone
Calcified trabecula
Osteoblast
Capillary

epiphysis fuses and the growth plate is eliminated. Epiphyseal fusion occurs at an earlier age in females than in males. Long bones also grow in diameter through a process of appositional growth beneath the periosteal surface.

Bone formation in the plate-like bones, such as the skull, facial bones, and scapula, occurs by intramembranous ossification. In these bones, there is direct mineralization of vascular connective tissue. Mesenchymal cells differentiate into osteoblasts and osteoid matrix is produced, converting mesenchyme into bone.

The process of bone remodeling is another critical element in the maintenance of bone health.[3] Throughout life, bone is continually being modified and renewed by the process of turnover. The remodeling cycle of formation and resorption continually replaces old bone with new, and repairs microdamage that is critical to skeletal integrity. In growing children, modeling is predominant with bone formation occurring at a greater rate and independent of bone resorption. This results in increases in bone mass and modification of bone shape.

Skeletal growth is directly affected by three primary hormonal systems—the pituitary-thyroid axis, the gonadal axis, and the growth hormone (GH)/insulin-like growth factor (IGF) system—as well as by paracrine function through different growth factors. GH is secreted by the anterior pituitary gland, and the rate of GH secretion is driven by GH-releasing factor from the medial hypothalamus. GH stimulates the release of IGF-1 at its sites of action. The result of increased GH/IGF activity is increased proliferation of epiphyseal chondrocytes, which stimulates linear growth. The gonadal and thyroid hormones appear to participate in both the proliferation and maturation of the growth plate. There is indirect evidence indicating that androgens are more important in chondrocyte proliferation, with estrogen and thyroid hormones more involved in the induction of epiphyseal fusion.[4]

Recent studies have provided evidence for the role of the parathyroid axis (PTHrP and PTH/PTHrP receptor) in chondrocyte differentiation and bone growth that may be an additional mechanism for disruption of normal growth in children with CKD.[5] Growth factors, such as BMP-7 or others may also play a role in the regulation of chondrocyte activity.

BONE MINERAL ACCRETION AND PEAK BONE MASS

Skeletal calcium accretion is a critical component of the dramatic increase in bone mass that occurs during childhood and adolescence, and is dependent on adequate levels of extracellular calcium and phosphorus for osteoid mineralization. The peak bone mass implies that optimal skeletal development during childhood and adolescence will prevent fractures in late adulthood.[6;7] This concept should, however, be related to body height and bone size.[8]

While limited data are available, it is likely that CKD during childhood compromises bone mineral accretion and results in reduced peak bone mass. Disturbances in calcitriol production and secondary hyperparathyroidism (SHPT) are likely to impact bone mass. Adequate calcitriol levels are critical to the availability of calcium. Increased levels of calcitriol have been shown to correspond with the increased skeletal calcium accumulation that occurs during puberty.[9] Elevated PTH levels result in increased resorption on the periosteal and endosteal surfaces that can compromise bone density, strength, and dimensions.

GROWTH DISTURBANCES IN CKD

Growth impairment is a common complication in children with CKD and is a significant obstacle to full rehabilitation. Skeletal growth can be assessed by comparing linear growth (height) to age- and sex-matched control values, or from the rate or velocity of bone growth over a defined period. In a study of 3,000 patients by the North American Pediatric Renal Transplant Cooperative, the mean height standard deviation scores (SDS) at the initiation of dialysis were 1.64 below the age- and sex-matched height levels.[10] Males and younger patients had greater growth impairment. A mean height SDS of -1.91 was found at the time of transplant in more than 6,600 patients evaluated. As the principal site of longitudinal bone growth, the epiphyseal growth plate is of primary interest when evaluating growth retardation in uremia. There are numerous factors that contribute to growth retardation in children with CKD, including metabolic acidosis, calcitriol deficiency, SHPT, inadequate protein and calorie intake, steroid therapy, anemia, hypogonadism during puberty, and—most importantly—disturbances in the IGF/GH system.

Metabolic Acidosis

Metabolic acidosis is a common component of kidney failure. It is often present in early CKD (Stages 2 and 3) and progresses in prevalence and severity as GFR declines. Persistent acidosis has been linked to delayed linear growth in children with renal tubular acidosis.[10;11] Acidosis may blunt linear growth by reducing renal tubular synthesis of calcitriol or by directly altering bone mineralization, although the primary mechanism is likely an inhibition of the GH/IGF-I axis.[12;13] Correction of acidosis by means of bicarbonate administration resulted in accelerated growth velocity and attainment of normal height in children with renal tubular acidosis and normal kidney function.[11]

While there are minimal direct clinical data to support the premise that correction of acidosis improves growth or bone disease in children with CKD, it has been recommended that total CO_2 levels be monitored regularly and that levels be maintained ≥ 22 mEq/L (22 mmol/L) in children over 2 years of age and ≥ 20 mEq/L in children under age 2. Oral alkali therapy or higher sodium bicarbonate dialysate concentration should be employed to maintain total plasma CO_2 above these levels.[14]

Insulin growth factor (IGF) and growth hormone (GH)

Resistance to GH and IGF-1 is postulated to be one of the principal factors in juvenile growth retardation in CKD.[15] Delayed growth occurs in children with CKD despite normal GH levels, or even in the presence of elevated GH levels that can occur with reduced renal clearance.[16] This disparity between growth and GH levels is evidence for resistance to GH at the target organs. Possible mechanisms for the reduced response to GH include diminished receptor expression or postreceptor defects, reductions in plasma GH-binding proteins, or elevated levels of IGF-binding protein (fragments) that have a high binding affinity for IGF-1, thereby reducing its bioavailability.[17-20]

Parathyroid hormone (PTH)

The disturbances in parathyroid gland activity and PTH action that accompany CKD can result in significant alterations in bone architecture. Children with severe SHPT may develop lesions in the epiphyseal growth plate that interfere with endochondral bone formation and therefore contribute to impaired bone growth.[21] Significant abnormalities in the morphology of the growth plate have been observed in children with advanced osteitis fibrosa.[22]

In rats with renal failure, the severity of SHPT has been shown to alter the expression of biomarkers that indicate chondrocyte proliferation and differentiation. Recent studies have suggested a critical role for PTHrP and the PTHrp/PTH receptor in the regulation of endochondral bone formation.[23]

Calcitriol deficiency may play a role in growth retardation, based on the findings that daily calcitriol supplementation can improve linear growth in children with CKD; however, the mechanism for this relationship has not been established.[24;25] Other studies have failed to demonstrate a consistent increase in growth velocity or linear growth in children with CKD who were treated with calcitriol.[25;26] While active vitamin D sterols may have a direct effect on growth, the primary mechanism of action is correction of SHPT and high-turnover bone lesions, thus improving growth plate function. However, at least *in vitro*, there is an interaction between the calcitropic and somatotropic hormone axis[27-29] and *in vivo*, a correlation between PTH sensitivity and growth hormone has been reported.[30] PTH responsiveness to hypocalcemic and hypercalcemic stimuli improved after GH replacement in adults with GH deficiency.[30]

Disturbances of Bone Remodeling in CKD

Numerous factors may contribute to disturbances in bone remodeling that accompany CKD, including abnormalities in PTH secretion and metabolism, vitamin D deficiency, imbalances in calcium and phosphorus metabolism, acid-base abnormalities, diminished PTH/PTHrp expression, and accumulation of aluminum. The spectrum of skeletal disorders in this population ranges from high-turnover lesions of SHPT to low-turnover lesions that accompany osteomalacia and adynamic bone (see Chapter 3). Most children with CKD or those on maintenance dialysis have some form of ROD.

The spectrum of ROD has been well characterized in children and adults treated with dialysis.[31-33] In adults, low-turnover osteodystrophy has become the most common skeletal lesion, with as many as 40% of adult patients on hemodialysis and 50% of continuous ambulatory peritoneal dialysis (CAPD) patients having bone biopsy evidence of adynamic bone.[34] In contrast, high-turnover/hyperparathyroid bone lesions remain the predominant lesion seen in pediatric CKD patients, despite the use of daily calcitriol therapy.[31-33] Adynamic bone affects only 15%-20% of pediatric patients treated with dialysis.[31;33]

Both high and low turnover of bone might have negative consequences. Recent studies have found an association among adynamic bone and higher fracture rates,[35] greater degree of arterial calcification,[36] and more severe growth retardation in children who developed adynamic bone after intermittent calcitriol administration and calcium-based binders.[37] Factors contributing to the development of adynamic bone include excess calcium intake from large doses of calcium-containing phosphate binders or high dialysate calcium concentrations, therapy with active vitamin D sterols, diabetes mellitus, parathyroidectomy, aging, and treatment with corticosteroids. [38] The incidence of low-turnover bone disease secondary to aluminum accumulation has been significantly reduced over the last decade.[39]

CLINICAL MANIFESTATIONS

In addition to the growth retardation and bone-turnover abnormalities described earlier, there are numerous specific and nonspecific manifestations of bone disease in children with CKD. These include slipped epiphyses, skeletal deformities, bone pain, muscle weakness, and extraskeletal calcifications (see Table 1).

TABLE 1. SIGNS AND SYMPTOMS OF BONE DISEASE IN CHILDREN WITH CKD

Metabolic Abnormalities
Hypocalcemia
Hyperphosphatemia
Hormonal Abnormalities
Altered vitamin D metabolism
Secondary hyperparathyroidism
Radiographic Abnormalities
Subperiosteal resorption
Osteosclerosis
Bone Disease
Linear growth failure
Delayed skeletal maturation and epiphyseal closure
Slipped epiphyses
Skeletal deformities resembling vitamin D-deficient rickets (genu valgum & genu varum, ankle valgus)
Avascular necrosis
Spontaneous tendon rupture
Meniscal tears
Bone pain
Fractures
Proximal Myopathy
Progressive muscle weakness, waddling gait
Extraskeletal (soft-tissue) Calcification
Calcification of blood vessels, lung, kidney, myocardium, coronary arteries and cardiac valves
Ocular Disease
Band keratopathy
Corneal calcification
Dermatological Disease
Pruritus
Skin ulceration and soft-tissue necrosis

Slipped epiphyses

Slipped epiphyses commonly occur in children with CKD. The most frequent location is the proximal femur, but slips have been reported in the distal radius and ulna, distal femur, proximal humerus, and distal tibia and fibula.[40-42] The upper and lower femoral epiphyses are most often affected in preschool children, with the upper femur and radial-ulnar epiphyses more often affected in older children. SHPT is likely the primary cause of slipped epiphyses in CKD. Higher PTH levels and severe osteitis fibrosa have been found to correlate with endosteal erosion and fibrosis and increased risk for slipped epiphyses.[42] Clinical symptoms associated with epiphysiolysis include limping, knee pain, waddling gait, limited range of motion, and limited ambulation. Possible sequelae of slipped epiphyses include severe varus deformity, osteonecrosis, chondrolysis, and degenerative joint disease. Definitive diagnosis is made by radiographs. Most slips can be stabilized with medical treatment of the underlying bone disease, and reduced weight bearing and movement at the site.[40-42] If conservative therapy does not achieve prompt stabilization of a slipped upper femur epiphysis, surgical pinning may be indicated, but control of SHPT is mandatory before the performance of orthopedic surgery.[43]

Skeletal deformities

Skeletal deformities are a common complication of ROD in children with long-term CKD. Angular deformity of the weight-bearing bones is the most common musculoskeletal abnormality seen. Of these, genu valgum is the most frequent, although genu varum, ankle valgum or varum, and coxa vara may also be seen.[40]

Deformities similar to vitamin D-deficient rickets are prevalent in children under age 4. These skeletal abnormalities include enlargement of the wrists and ankles due to metaphysis widening, rachitic rosary, Harrison grooves and craniotabes.[44] In children under age 10 with high bone-growth velocity, abnormalities are commonly seen in long bones, particularly the lower extremities.[45] Other skeletal abnormalities seen include psuedoclubbing, ulnar deviation, pes varus, and dental abnormalities. The first step in correcting these deformities is to treat the underlying metabolic bone disease, mainly SHPT. If the deformity does not resolve with medical therapy, surgical intervention may be required; indeed, up to 30% of children with CKD have required corrective orthopedic procedures.[46] Controlling hyperparathyroidism both before and after surgical procedures is critical to bone healing.

Musculoskeletal symptoms

Nonspecific symptoms such as bone pain, muscle cramps during repetitive motion activities, and proximal myopathy that limit activities of daily living are common manifestations of pediatric ROD. The mechanism for muscle weakness is poorly understood. Contributing factors likely include SHPT, aluminum bone disease, phosphate depletion, and vitamin D deficiency. Improvement in muscle strength has been attributed to calcitriol treatment.[47]

Extraskeletal calcification

A number of recent studies have identified an association between abnormalities of bone and mineral metabolism, and the development of vascular calcifications and increased mortality in patients with CKD (see Chapters 4 and 5). In a postmortem analysis of clinical, biochemical, and autopsy data in 120 children with CKD, soft-tissue and vascular calcification was associated with use of active vitamin D sterols and calcium-based phosphate binders.[48] Young adults with childhood-onset CKD have significantly higher levels of coronary artery calcification than age matched controls. Inflammation (indicated by increased C-reactive protein) elevated plasma phosphorus and calcium-phosphorus product (CaXP), high total calcium intake, and elevated PTH levels all have positive correlations with vascular calcification found in childhood-onset CKD.[49;50] Accurate diagnosis and optimal treatment of the abnormalities in bone and mineral metabolism may play a critical role in reducing the accelerated vascular calcification in children with CKD and thereby minimize cardiovascular mortality.

THERAPEUTIC CONSIDERATIONS

As in the adult population, the management of ROD in pediatric CKD includes measures to normalize calcium and phosphorus levels and maintain PTH within an acceptable range, while preventing extraskeletal and vascular calcifications and maximizing bone health (see Chapter 6). In addition, correction of acidosis, treatment of anemia, and nutrition counseling are important elements to improve growth and maximize bone health in children with CKD.[51]

Treatment considerations unique to pediatrics include measures that promote normal maturation and growth of the skeletal system, and prevent the development of bone deformities and the process of vascular calcification. This includes administration of recombinant human growth hormone (rhGH) and control of SHPT through appropriate use of vitamin D sterols and phosphate binders.

Growth hormone

Pharmacological doses of rhGH improve linear growth in children with growth failure secondary to CKD.[52-54] This therapy is effective in CKD Stage 3 and 4, without adversely affecting GFR.[52;54] The rate of growth diminishes after the first year of therapy, yet continues to be higher than before treatment.[52] Long-term therapy with rhGH in children with CKD has the potential to allow attainment of target adult height.[15]

Treatment with rhGH appears to be more effective in CKD Stage 3 and 4 than when initiated in children on maintenance dialysis.[55] The cause of this disparity in effectiveness of rhGH is not clear, but may be related to concurrent therapy with active vitamin D sterols during dialysis, or a progressive insensitivity to GH as uremia progresses.[55] Initiating rhGH earlier in the course of CKD provides a higher probability of growth normalization.

It has been recommended that rhGH therapy be considered in all children on dialysis with growth potential, under the conditions detailed below.[14;15]

Therapy may be appropriate in children who have:

- height for chronological age more negative than 2.0 SDS or
- height velocity for chronological age more negative than 2.0 SDS;
- growth potential documented by open epiphyses; and
- no other contraindication for recombinant hGH use.

Prior to considering the use of rhGH, there should be correction of:

- insufficient intake of energy, protein and other nutrients;
- acidosis;
- hyperphosphatemia (the level of plasma phosphorus should be less than 1.5 times the upper limit of normal for age); and
- SHPT.

Acidosis and/or severe hyperphosphatemia can impair the action of rhGH. It is therefore essential to correct the acidosis and control the plasma phosphorus levels prior to initiating rhGH therapy. Therapy with rhGH can increase PTH levels, thereby worsening SHPT.[56] In general, rhGH therapy is suggested not to be started until iPTH levels are no greater than 2X the target upper limit for CKD Stages 2-4 (see Table 2) or 1.5X [450 pg/ml (49.5 pmol/L)] the target upper limit in CKD Stage 5.

TABLE 2. TARGET iPTH RANGE IN CHILDREN BASED ON CKD STAGE[59]

CKD Stage	GFR Range (mL/min/1.73 m²)	Target iPTH
2	60-89	35-70 pg/mL (3.9-7.7 pmol/L)
3	30-59	35-70 pg/mL (3.9-7.7 pmol/L)
4	15-29	70-110 pg/mL (7.7-12.1 pmol/L)
5	<15 or dialysis	200-300 pg/mL (22-33 pmol/L)

Abbreviations: CKD, chronic kidney disease; GFR, glomerular filtration rate; iPTH, intact parathyroid hormone

GH therapy may increase the risk for slipped epiphysis.[57;58] In children with CKD, who already have an inherent predisposition for bone disease and slipped epiphyses, vigilant screening is recommended. Hip and wrist X-rays may be evaluated to rule out slipped epiphyses or other skeletal deformities, and these problems should be corrected prior to starting rhGH.

It is recommended that patients receiving rhGH be monitored closely, including serial radiographs and regular evaluation of calcium, phosphorus, and PTH. Patients who develop severe SHPT may have rhGH therapy discontinued until PTH levels are reduced. Increased use of vitamin D sterols to control SHPT may be required in patients receiving rhGH.[56] Therapy should be discontinued if a patient develops a slipped capital femoral epiphysis or symptoms related to high-turnover bone disease. GH therapy may be discontinued permanently once the epiphyses have closed.

The recommended dose of rhGH, which is given as a daily subcutaneous injection, is 0.05 mg/kg/day or 30 IU/m²/week.[14] If the patient does not respond to rhGH after 12 months of treatment (e.g., increase of growth velocity by <2 cm/year), discontinuation should be considered. Prior to discontinuation, a thorough evaluation of the patient is suggested to ensure that other causes of growth retardation in children with CKD have been corrected. If the patient reaches the 50th percentile for target height following rhGH treatment, it is advisable to discontinue rhGH treatment and monitor the patient. If the height SDS decreases by 0.25 during a subsequent observation period, it is advisable to consider reinstitution of the rhGH therapy.

Secondary hyperparathyroidism

As renal function diminishes with CKD, calcitriol levels decrease progressively. This leads to reduced intestinal absorption of calcium and eventually hypocalcemia, which can impair the normal suppression of the pre-pro-PTH gene that initiates the synthesis of PTH. The progressive decline in GFR also leads to phosphorus retention and hyperphosphatemia. Hypocalcemia, hyperphosphatemia, and decreased calcitriol levels lead to the development of SHPT (see Chapter 3). As previously discussed, SHPT has a significant impact on both bone remodeling and growth; therefore, therapeutic measures to normalize PTH levels are critical to successful management of children with CKD.

The first step in treating SHPT is to control elevated phosphorus levels according to the stage of CKD. For children with kidney failure (CKD Stage 5), including those treated with hemodialysis or peritoneal dialysis, the plasma level of phosphorus is recommended to be maintained between 3.5-5.5 mg/dL (1.12-1.76 mmol/L) during adolescence and between 4-6 mg/dL (1.28-1.92 mmol/L) for children between the ages of 1-12 years. In children with CKD Stages 2-4, plasma phosphorus levels are recommended to be maintained within the normal range for age. For children with plasma phosphorus levels above these ranges, dietary phosphorus restriction may be beneficial as long as it does not compromise overall nutrition. If phosphorus remains elevated despite dietary modification, phosphate binder therapy is recommended. In infants and young children, calcium-based binders are preferred. In older children and adolescents either calcium- or noncalcium-based binders can be used. In general the total intake of calcium from the diet and calcium-based phosphate binders should not exceed two times the age-specific daily recommended intake.[59] Calcium-free and metal-free phosphate binders are preferred in the presence of elevated calcium or CaXP. The calcium-free, metal-free, phosphate binder sevelamer hydrochloride has been used in pediatric nephrology for several years and it has been shown to be effective and well tolerated in children.[60;61] Lanthanum carbonate is another calcium-free binder that has been shown to be effective in reducing phosphorus in adult dialysis patients.[62;63] Lanthanum is a rare earth metal with the potential to accumulate in various tissues.[64] It has not been studied in children, and concerns remain regarding its long-term use in children because lanthanum has been shown to bind to chondroitin sulfate (a critical component of cartilage and, therefore, the growth plate.)[65] Consequently, it cannot be recommended for use in children until further studies have been performed that exclude this potential toxicity.

Increasing the dose of dialysis may also be an effective tool to treat persistent hyperphosphatemia. If hyperphosphatemia (plasma phosphorus >7.0 mg/dL [2.24 mmol/L]) is resistant to other phosphate binders and increasing the dialysis dose is not an option, a single, short-term (4-6 weeks) course of an aluminum-based phosphate binder may be considered.[59] If aluminum-based binders are used, therapy with sodium citrate must be discontinued because citrate enhances intestinal aluminum absorption. If correction of acidosis is required, sodium bicarbonate therapy can be given in combination with aluminum hydroxide.[66]

Corrected levels of total plasma calcium should be maintained within the normal range. If PTH remains elevated (Table 2) despite normalization of calcium and attempts to manage phosphorus, then treatment with vitamin D may be considered. In CKD Stages 2-4, the plasma level of 25-hydroxyvitamin D (25OHD), the substrate for the kidney's generation of the active vitamin D hormone, is a good measure of vitamin D status. If plasma 25OHD levels are <30 ng/mL (75 nmol/L), the initial therapy for SHPT is oral ergocalciferol (Table 3).[59] Calcium and phosphorus should be monitored during therapy. If 25OHD levels are >30 ng/mL (75 nmol/L), an active vitamin D sterol may be considered to treat SHPT (Table 4).

TABLE 3. RECOMMENDED SUPPLEMENTATION FOR VITAMIN D DEFICIENCY/INSUFFICIENCY IN CHILDREN WITH CKD STAGES 3 AND 4[59]

Serum 25(OH)D (ng/mL)	Definition	Ergocalciferol Dose (Vitamin D$_2$)	Duration (months)	Comment
<5	Severe vitamin D deficiency	8,000 IU (200 µg) per day orally or 50,000 IU (1,250 µg) per week X 4 weeks; then 4,000 IU (100 µg) per day or 50,000 IU (1,250 µg) per month for 2 months	3 months	Measure 25(OH)D levels after 3 months
5-15	Mild vitamin D deficiency	4,000 IU (100 µg) per day orally or 50,000 IU (1,250 µg) every other week for 12 weeks	3 months	Measure 25(OH)D levels after 3 months
16-30	Vitamin D insufficiency	2,000 IU (50 µg) per day orally or 50,000 IU (1,250 µg) every 4 weeks for 12 weeks	3 months	Measure 25(OH)D levels after 3 months

Abbreviation: CKD, chronic kidney disease.

TABLE 4. PLASMA LEVELS OF iPTH, CALCUIM, AND PHOSPHATE REQUIRED FOR INITIATION OF ORAL VITAMIN D STEROL THERAPY, AND RECOMMENDED INITIAL DOSES IN CHILDREN WITH STAGES STAGES 2-4 CKD[59]

Plasma iPTH	Plasma Ca	Plasma P	Dose Oral Calcitriol
CKD Stages 2 and 3: >70 pg/mL (7.7 pmol/L)	≤ <10 mg/dL (2.5 mmol/L)	age-appropriate levels	<10 kg: 0.05 µg every other day
CKD Stage 4: >110 pg/mL (12.1 pmol/L)			10-20 kg: 0.1-0.15 µg/day
			>20 kg: 0.25 µg/day

Abbreviations: Ca, calcium; CKD, chronic kidney disease; iPTH, intact parathyroid hormone; P, phosphorus.

In patients with CKD Stage 5, an active vitamin D sterol will be needed and may be considered in children with intact PTH levels >300 pg/mL (33 pmol/L) (Table 5).[59] Treatment with calcitriol or another vitamin D sterol (such as paricalcitol or doxercalciferol) is effective in reducing elevated PTH levels, ameliorating bone pain and muscle weakness, and can improve the histological bone abnormalities that accompany severe hyperparathyroidism.[61;67] Both daily oral and intermittent, high-dose calcitriol therapy have been used to reduce elevated PTH levels in children with SHPT. However, the effect on bone appears to vary depending on the dosage, frequency, and route of administration. Despite treatment with vitamin D sterols, high-turnover/hyperparathyroid bone disease remains the predominant bone lesion in dialyzed children.[68;69] When children with biopsy-proven, high-turnover bone disease were followed for 1 year while on daily calcitriol therapy, bone lesions of SHPT persisted or progressed in the vast majority of the patients.[70] On the other hand, therapy with intermittent calcitriol combined with calcium-containing phosphate binders corrected many of the histological features of high-bone turnover disease in a cohort of pediatric patients. However, a substantial proportion of children developed adynamic bone disease, despite persistently elevated PTH levels.[2] Patients with adynamic bone are more prone to hypercalcemia, which may be associated with increased mortality. Based on these findings, intermittent dosing of vitamin D sterols— whether by the oral, intravenous, or intraperitoneal route—may be preferable. In order to minimize the potential for adynamic bone in CKD Stage 5 patients, the dose of active vitamin D sterol should be adjusted to maintain a plasma PTH level >200 pg/mL (22 pmol/L). More recently, the intermittent administration of active oral vitamin D sterols (calcitriol/doxercalciferol) in combination with either calcium-based binders or sevelamer was shown to prevent the development of adynamic bone by adjusting the dose of active vitamin D sterols to maintain PTH levels between 300-400 pg/ml (33-44 pmol/L).[61] Furthermore, therapy with sevelamer allowed the use of higher doses of active vitamin D sterols with concomitant reductions in PTH levels, without leading to increments in plasma calcium concentrations.[61]

TABLE 5. INITIAL CALCITRIOL DOSING RECOMMENDATIONS FOR CHILDREN ON MAINTENANCE DIALYSIS[59]

iPTH (pg/mL) [pmol/L]	Plasma Ca (mg/dL) [mmol/L]	Plasma P (mg/dL) [mmol/L]	CaxP product*	Calcitriol dose per HD session (TIW)	Calcitriol dose for patients receiving PD (TIW) [2;70]
300-500 [33-55]	<10 [2.5]	<5.5 [1.76] for adolescents <6.5 [2.08] for infants and children	<55 for adolescents <65 for infants and children	0.0075µg/kg/HD (maximum = 0.25 µg)	0.0075 µg/kg/HD (maximum = 0.25 µg)
500-1,000 [55-110]	<10 [2.5]	<5.5 [1.76] for adolescents <6.5 [2.08] for infants and children	<55 for adolescents <65 for infants and children	0.015 µg/kg/HD (maximum = 0.5 µg)	0.015 µg/kg/HD (maximum = 0.5 µg)
>1,000 [110]	<10.5 [2.63]	<5.5 [1.76] for adolescents <6.5 [2.08] for infants and children	<55 for adolescents <65 for infants and children	0.025 µg/kg/HD (maximum = 1 µg)	0.025 µg/kg/HD (maximum = 1 µg)

* <65 in children below 12 years of age

Abbreviations: Ca, calcium; CKD, chronic kidney disease; HD, hemodialysis; iPTH, intact parathyroid hormone; P, phosphorus; PD, peritoneal dialysis; TIW, thrice weekly.

Findings related to the role of vitamin D therapy in improving growth potential in children are inconsistent. Several investigators have demonstrated improvements in growth in children with CKD during treatment with active D sterols.[24;25] Other recent studies have, however, failed to show that 1,25(OH)$_2$D therapy provides consistent improvement in linear growth.[26;32;71] Large, intermittent doses of calcitriol may even diminish linear growth in prepubertal children with adynamic bone.[37] Further studies are needed to determine optimal PTH levels associated with maximal growth velocity when vitamin D and rhGH are administered independently and in combination.

Other important considerations to maximize bone health and promote normal development in this population include exercise and resistance training, adequate treatment of anemia, maximizing nutritional status, correction of acidosis, vigilant monitoring for bone deformities, and orthopedic referral when appropriate. Many pediatric CKD patients will undergo kidney transplantation. In addition to the pre-existing bone and mineral abnormalities, there are a number of skeletal changes unique to the post-transplant period (see Chapter 7). Maintaining bone health following transplant is critical to maximize rehabilitation and normal growth and development, and to prevent the development of vascular calcifications in these children.

CONCLUSIONS

Metabolic bone disease is a significant clinical problem in children with CKD. The pathophysiological mechanisms underlying the abnormalities in bone and mineral metabolism that accompany uremia are similar in adults and children. However, there are distinct differences in the clinical manifestations of renal bone disease in children, primarily due to the active growth state of the skeleton. The present chapter describes the specific pathophysiological mechanisms of renal osteodystrophy in children, and the clinical manifestations of this disorder. General therapeutic recommendations for the treatment of children with CKD and ROD are based on the available evidence; however, further studies in children are necessary to develop individualized treatment plans.

REFERENCES

*1. Groothoff JW, Offringa M, Eck-Smit BL, Gruppen MP, Van De Kar NJ, Wolff ED, Lilien MR, Davin JC, Heymans HS, Dekker FW: Severe bone disease and low bone mineral density after juvenile renal failure. Kidney Int 63:266-275, 2003

*2. Salusky IB, Kuizon BD, Belin TR, Ramirez JA, Gales B, Segre GV, Goodman WG: Intermittent calcitriol therapy in secondary hyperparathyroidism: a comparison between oral and intraperitoneal administration. Kidney Int 54:907-914, 1998

3. Baron R: Anatomy and ultrastructure of bone, in Favus MJ (ed): Primer on the metabolic bone diseases and disorders of mineral metabolism, chap 1. Philadelphia, PA, 1999, pp 3-10

4. Smith EP, Boyd J, Frank GR, Takahashi H, Cohen RM, Specker B, Williams TC, Lubahn DB, Korach KS: Estrogen resistance caused by a mutation in the estrogen-receptor gene in a man. N Engl J Med 331:1056-1061, 1994

5. Kuizon BD, Salusky IB: Growth retardation in children with chronic renal failure. J Bone Miner Res 14:1680-1690, 1999

6. Chan GM, Hoffman K, McMurry M: Effects of dairy products on bone and body composition in pubertal girls. J Pediatr 126:551-556, 1995

7. Goulding A, Jones IE, Taylor RW, Manning PJ, Williams SM: More broken bones: a 4-year double cohort study of young girls with and without distal forearm fractures. J Bone Miner Res 15:2011-2018, 2000

*8. Schonau E: The peak bone mass concept: is it still relevant? Pediatr Nephrol 19:825-831, 2004

9. Aksnes L, Aarskog D: Plasma concentrations of vitamin D metabolites in puberty: effect of sexual maturation and implications for growth. J Clin Endocrinol Metab 55:94-101, 1982

10. Furth SL, Hwang W, Yang C, Neu AM, Fivush BA, Powe NR: Growth failure, risk of hospitalization and death for children with end-stage renal disease. Pediatr Nephrol 17:450-455, 2002

11. McSherry E, Morris RC, Jr.: Attainment and maintenance of normal stature with alkali therapy in infants and children with classic renal tubular acidosis. J Clin Invest 61:509-527, 1978

12. Challa A, Krieg RJ, Jr., Thabet MA, Veldhuis JD, Chan JC: Metabolic acidosis inhibits growth hormone secretion in rats: mechanism of growth retardation. Am J Physiol 265:E547-E553, 1993

13. Kuemmerle N, Krieg RJ, Jr., Latta K, Challa A, Hanna JD, Chan JC: Growth hormone and insulin-like growth factor in non-uremic acidosis and uremic acidosis. Kidney Int Suppl 58:S102-S105, 1997

14. National Kidney Foundation.: National kidney foundation K/DOQI clinical practice guidelines for nutrition in chronic renal failure. Am J Kidney Dis 37:S66-S70, 2001

*15. Haffner D, Schaefer F, Nissel R, Wuhl E, Tonshoff B, Mehls O: Effect of growth hormone treatment on the adult height of children with chronic renal failure. German Study Group for Growth Hormone Treatment in Chronic Renal Failure. N Engl J Med 343:923-930, 2000

16. Tonshoff B, Cronin MJ, Reichert M, Haffner D, Wingen AM, Blum WF, Mehls O: Reduced concentration of serum growth hormone (GH)-binding protein in children with chronic renal failure: correlation with GH insensitivity. The European Study Group for Nutritional Treatment of Chronic Renal Failure in Childhood. The German Study Group for Growth Hormone Treatment in Chronic Renal Failure. J Clin Endocrinol Metab 82:1007-1013, 1997

17. Powell DR, Liu F, Baker BK, Hintz RL, Lee PD, Durham SK, Brewer ED, Frane JW, Watkins SL, Hogg RJ: Modulation of growth factors by growth hormone in children with chronic renal failure. The Southwest Pediatric Nephrology Study Group. Kidney Int 51:1970-1979, 1997

18. Schaefer F, Chen Y, Tsao T, Nouri P, Rabkin R: Impaired JAK-STAT signal transduction contributes to growth hormone resistance in chronic uremia. J Clin Invest 108:467-475, 2001

19. Tonshoff B, Eden S, Weiser E, Carlsson B, Robinson IC, Blum WF, Mehls O: Reduced hepatic growth hormone (GH) receptor gene expression and increased plasma GH binding protein in experimental uremia. Kidney Int 45:1085-1092, 1994

20. Tonshoff B, Blum WF, Mehls O: Derangements of the somatotropic hormone axis in chronic renal failure. Kidney Int Suppl 58:S106-S113, 1997

21. Mehls O, Ritz E: Renal Osteodystrophy, in Holliday M, Barratt T, Vernier R (eds): Pediatric Nephrology, chap 52. Baltimore, 1987, pp 852-879

22. Krempien B, Mehls O, Ritz E: Morphological studies on pathogenesis of epiphyseal slipping in uremic children. Virchows Arch A Pathol Anat Histol 362:129-143, 1974

23. Sanchez CP, Salusky IB, Kuizon BD, Abdella P, Juppner H, Goodman WG: Growth of long bones in renal failure: roles of hyperparathyroidism, growth hormone and calcitriol. Kidney Int 54:1879-1887, 1998

24. Chesney RW, Moorthy AV, Eisman JA, Jax DK, Mazess RB, DeLuca HF: Increased growth after long-term oral 1alpha,25-vitamin D3 in childhood renal osteodystrophy. N Engl J Med 298:238-242, 1978

*25. Langman CB, Mazur AT, Baron R, Norman ME: 25-hydroxyvitamin D3 (calcifediol) therapy of juvenile renal osteodystrophy: beneficial effect on linear growth velocity. J Pediatr 100:815-820, 1982

*26. Chan JC, McEnery PT, Chinchilli VM, Abitbol CL, Boineau FG, Friedman AL, Lum GM, Roy S, III, Ruley EJ, Strife CF: A prospective, double-blind study of growth failure in children with chronic renal insufficiency and the effectiveness of treatment with calcitriol versus dihydrotachysterol. The Growth Failure in Children with Renal Diseases Investigators. J Pediatr 124:520-528, 1994

27. Green J, Goldberg R, Maor G: PTH ameliorates acidosis-induced adverse effects in skeletal growth centers: the PTH-IGF-I axis. Kidney Int 63:487-500, 2003

28. Klaus G, Jux C, Leiber K, Hugel U, Mehls O: Interaction between insulin-like growth factor I, growth hormone, parathyroid hormone, 1 alpha,25-dihydroxyvitamin D3 and steroids on epiphyseal chondrocytes. Acta Paediatr Suppl 417:69-71, 1996

29. Yamaguchi M, Ogata N, Shinoda Y, Akune T, Kamekura S, Terauchi Y, Kadowaki T, Hoshi K, Chung UI, Nakamura K, Kawaguchi H: Insulin Receptor Substrate-1 Is Required for Bone Anabolic Function of Parathyroid Hormone in Mice. Endocrinology 2005

30. Ahmad AM, Thomas J, Clewes A, Hopkins MT, Guzder R, Ibrahim H, Durham BH, Vora JP, Fraser WD: Effects of growth hormone replacement on parathyroid hormone sensitivity and bone mineral metabolism. J Clin Endocrinol Metab 88:2860-2868, 2003

31. Mathias R, Salusky I, Harman W, Paredes A, Emans J, Segre G, Goodman W: Renal bone disease in pediatric and young adult patients on hemodialysis in a children's hospital. J Am Soc Nephrol 3:1938-1946, 1993

32. Salusky IB, Coburn JW, Brill J, Foley J, Slatopolsky E, Fine RN, Goodman WG: Bone disease in pediatric patients undergoing dialysis with CAPD or CCPD. Kidney Int 33:975-982, 1988

33. Salusky IB, Ramirez JA, Oppenheim W, Gales B, Segre GV, Goodman WG: Biochemical markers of renal osteodystrophy in pediatric patients undergoing CAPD/CCPD. Kidney Int 45:253-258, 1994

34. Sherrard DJ, Hercz G, Pei Y, Maloney NA, Greenwood C, Manuel A, Saiphoo C, Fenton SS, Segre GV: The spectrum of bone disease in end-stage renal failure—an evolving disorder. Kidney Int 43:436-442, 1993

35. Coco M, Rush H: Increased incidence of hip fractures in dialysis patients with low serum parathyroid hormone. Am J Kidney Dis 36:1115-1121, 2000

36. London GM, Marty C, Marchais SJ, Guerin AP, Metivier F, de Vernejoul MC: Arterial calcifications and bone histomorphometry in end-stage renal disease. J Am Soc Nephrol 15:1943-1951, 2004

37. Kuizon BD, Goodman WG, Juppner H, Boechat I, Nelson P, Gales B, Salusky IB: Diminished linear growth during intermittent calcitriol therapy in children undergoing CCPD. Kidney Int 53:205-211, 1998

38. Salusky IB, Goodman WG: Adynamic renal osteodystrophy: Is there a problem? J Am Soc Nephrol 12:1978-1985, 2001

39. Hercz G, Pei Y, Greenwood C, Manuel A, Saiphoo C, Goodman WG, Segre GV, Fenton S, Sherrard DJ: Aplastic osteodystrophy without aluminum: the role of "suppressed" parathyroid function. Kidney Int 44:860-866, 1993

40. Barrett IR, Papadimitriou DG: Skeletal disorders in children with renal failure. J Pediatr Orthop 16:264-272, 1996

41. Loder RT, Hensinger RN: Slipped capital femoral epiphysis associated with renal failure osteodystrophy. J Pediatr Orthop 17:205-211, 1997

42. Mehls O, Ritz E, Krempien B, Gilli G, Link K, Willich E, Scharer K: Slipped epiphyses in renal osteodystrophy. Arch Dis Child 50:545-554, 1975

43. Oppenheim WL, Bowen RE, McDonough PW, Funahashi TT, Salusky IB: Outcome of slipped capital femoral epiphysis in renal osteodystrophy. J Pediatr Orthop 23:169-174, 2003

44. Mehls O: Renal osteodystrohy in children: etiology and clinical aspects, in Fine RN, Gruskin AB (eds): End stage renal disease in children, Philadelphia, 1984, pp 227-250

45. Davids JR, Fisher R, Lum G, Von Glinski S: Angular deformity of the lower extremity in children with renal osteodystrophy. J Pediatr Orthop 12:291-299, 1992

46. Sanchez CP, Salusky I: Bone and mineral metabolism in children with chronic renal failure, in Bushinsky D (ed): Renal osteodystrophy, chap 15. Philadelphia, 1998, pp 381-402

47. Henderson RG, Russell RG, Ledingham JG, Smith R, Oliver DO, Walton RJ, Small DG, Preston C, Warner GT: Effects of 1,25-dihydroxycholecalciferol on calcium absorption, muscle weakness, and bone disease in chronic renal failure. Lancet 1:379-384, 1974

*48. Milliner DS, Zinsmeister AR, Lieberman E, Landing B: Soft tissue calcification in pediatric patients with end-stage renal disease. Kidney Int 38:931-936, 1990

*49. Oh J, Wunsch R, Turzer M, Bahner M, Raggi P, Querfeld U, Mehls O, Schaefer F: Advanced coronary and carotid arteriopathy in young adults with childhood-onset chronic renal failure. Circulation 106:100-105, 2002

*50. Goodman WG, Goldin J, Kuizon BD, Yoon C, Gales B, Sider D, Wang Y, Chung J, Emerick A, Greaser L, Elashoff RM, Salusky IB: Coronary-artery calcification in young adults with end-stage renal disease who are undergoing dialysis. N Engl J Med 342:1478-1483, 2000

51. Van Dyck M, Bilem N, Proesmans W: Conservative treatment for chronic renal failure from birth: a 3-year follow-up study. Pediatr Nephrol 13:865-869, 1999

52. Fine RN, Kohaut EC, Brown D, Perlman AJ: Growth after recombinant human growth hormone treatment in children with chronic renal failure: report of a multicenter randomized double-blind placebo-controlled study. Genentech Cooperative Study Group. J Pediatr 124:374-382, 1994

53. Hokken-Koelega AC, Stijnen T, de Muinck Keizer-Schrama SM, Wit JM, Wolff ED, de Jong MC, Donckerwolcke RA, Abbad NC, Bot A, Blum WF: Placebo-controlled, double-blind, cross-over trial of growth hormone treatment in prepubertal children with chronic renal failure. Lancet 338:585-590, 1991

54. Mehls O, Broyer M: Growth response to recombinant human growth hormone in short prepubertal children with chronic renal failure with or without dialysis. The European/Australian Study Group. Acta Paediatr Suppl 399:81-87, 1994

55. Wuhl E, Haffner D, Nissel R, Schaefer F, Mehls O: Short dialyzed children respond less to growth hormone than patients prior to dialysis. German Study Group for Growth Hormone Treatment in Chronic Renal Failure. Pediatr Nephrol 10:294-298, 1996

56. Sieniawska M, Panczyk-Tomaszewska M, Ziolkowska H: The influence of growth hormone treatment on bone metabolism in dialysis patients. Br J Clin Pract Suppl 85:61-63, 1996

57. Prasad V, Greig F, Bastian W, Castells S, Juan C, AvRuskin TW: Slipped capital femoral epiphysis during treatment with recombinant growth hormone for isolated, partial growth hormone deficiency. J Pediatr 116:397-399, 1990

58. Watkins SL: Bone disease in patients receiving growth hormone. Kidney Int Suppl 53:S126-S127, 1996

59. National Kidney Foundation. National kidney foundation K/DOQI clinical practice guidelines for bone metabolism and disease in children with chronic kidney disease. Am J Kidney Dis., 2005. Ref Type: In Press

60. Mahdavi H, Kuizon BD, Gales B, Wang HJ, Elashoff RM, Salusky IB: Sevelamer hydrochloride: an effective phosphate binder in dialyzed children. Pediatr Nephrol 18:1260-1264, 2003

61. Salusky IB, Goodman WG, Sahney S, Gales B, Perilloux A, Wang HJ, Elashoff RM, Juppner H: Sevelamer Controls Parathyroid Hormone-Induced Bone Disease as Efficiently as Calcium Carbonate without Increasing Serum Calcium Levels during Therapy with Active Vitamin D Sterols. J Am Soc Nephrol 16:2501-2508, 2005

62. D'Haese PC, Spasovski GB, Sikole A, Hutchison A, Freemont TJ, Sulkova S, Swanepoel C, Pejanovic S, Djukanovic L, Balducci A, Coen G, Sulowicz W, Ferreira A, Torres A, Curic S, Popovic M, Dimkovic N, De Broe ME: A multicenter study on the effects of lanthanum carbonate (Fosrenol) and calcium carbonate on renal bone disease in dialysis patients. Kidney Int Suppl S73-S78, 2003

63. Joy MS, Finn WF: Randomized, double-blind, placebo-controlled, dose-titration, phase III study assessing the efficacy and tolerability of lanthanum carbonate: a new phosphate binder for the treatment of hyperphosphatemia. Am J Kidney Dis 42:96-107, 2003

64. Lacour B, Lucas A, Auchere D, Ruellan N, Serre Patey NM, Drueke TB: Chronic renal failure is associated with increased tissue deposition of lanthanum after 28-day oral administration. Kidney Int 67:1062-1069, 2005

65. Harris AF, Cotty VF: The effect of lanthanum chloride and related compounds on calcification. Arch Int Pharmacodyn Ther 186:269-278, 1970

66. Coburn JW, Mischel MG, Goodman WG, Salusky IB: Calcium citrate markedly enhances aluminum absorption from aluminum hydroxide. Am J Kidney Dis 17:708-711, 1991

67. Hamdy NA, Kanis JA, Beneton MN, Brown CB, Juttmann JR, Jordans JG, Josse S, Meyrier A, Lins RL, Fairey IT: Effect of alfacalcidol on natural course of renal bone disease in mild to moderate renal failure. BMJ 310:358-363, 1995

68. Mathias RS, Salusky IB, Harmon WH, Paredes A, Emans J, Segre GV, Goodman WG: Renal bone disease in pediatric patients and young adults treated by hemodialysis in a childrens hospital. J Am Soc Nephrol 12:1938-1946, 1993

69. Salusky IB, Ramirez JA, Oppenheim WL, Gales B, Segre GV, Goodman WG: Biochemical markers of renal osteodystrophy in pediatric patients undergoing CAPD/CCPD. Kidney Int 45:253-258, 1994

70. Goodman WG, Salusky IB: Evolution of secondary hyperparathyroidism during oral calcitriol therapy in pediatric renal osteodystrophy. Contrib Nephrol 90:189-195, 1991

71. Hodson EM, Evans RA, Dunstan CR, Hills E, Wong SY, Rosenberg AR, Roy LP: Treatment of childhood renal osteodystrophy with calcitriol or ergocalciferol. Clin Nephrol 24:192-200, 1985

*Suggested Reading

OSTEOPOROSIS AND HYPOGONADISM IN CKD PATIENTS

José R. Weisinger
Mary B. Leonard

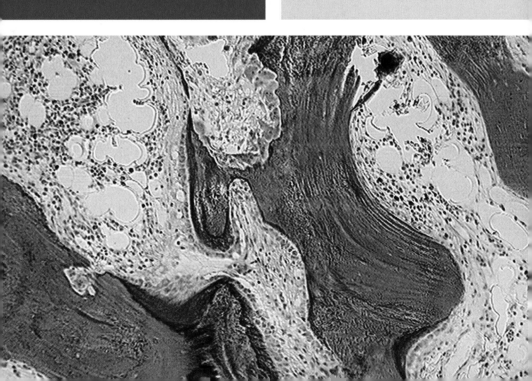

CHAPTER 9

OSTEOPOROSIS AND HYPOGONADISM IN CKD PATIENTS

José R. Weisinger and Mary B. Leonard

Compromised bone strength is a significant comorbidity in the chronic kidney disease (CKD) population. Dialysis patients have an increased risk of fracture and higher mortality rates associated with fractures.[1-3] Renal osteodystrophy (ROD) is the principal term used to describe the complex disorder of bone and mineral metabolism that compromises bone strength in CKD patients. Hypogonadism and osteoporosis receive less attention than secondary hyper-parathyroidism (SHPT) and bone-turnover abnormalities, but are still important components of the alterations in bone structure and function seen in CKD. This chapter will provide a review of the role of hypogonadism and related osteoporosis in the evolution of ROD, and discuss assessment and treatment considerations.

ROLE OF GONADAL STEROIDS IN BONE HEALTH

The gonadal steroids produced by the ovaries (estrogens) and testes (androgens) play an important role in skeletal maturation and maintenance of bone health. Sex differences in bone mass and dimensions are established during puberty. For example, cortical width increases by periosteal bone formation in boys, and by less periosteal bone formation but more endocorti-cal apposition in girls.[4] The greater periosteal apposition in males results in greater bone strength in bending and torsion. Androgens stimulate periosteal apposition while estrogens inhibit periosteal apposition and stimulate endosteal apposition during puberty.

The decrease in estrogen availability that occurs with aging and menopause is a primary cause of the progressive bone loss in postmenopausal women and a contributing cause of age-relat-ed bone loss in men.[5] Some data suggest that estrogens are more important than androgens in the development and maintenance of the male skeleton, as is the case in women.[6] Estrogen appears to be the dominant sex steroid in regulating bone resorption, whereas testosterone is more important for bone formation.[7] Receptors for both estrogen and testosterone have been identified in bone, but their exact mechanism of action is unclear.[8] Both hormones participate at some level in the regulation of bone formation and resorption (Table 1).

Estrogen, through its effect on local cytokine levels, inhibits bone osteoclast recruitment and activity. Low estrogen levels have been associated with increased osteoclastic activity and bone resorption.[9;10] Estrogen also may affect parathyroid hormone (PTH) activity by increasing PTH mRNA transcription in the parathyroid cells and by inhibiting the responsiveness of bone cells to the actions of PTH.[11;12]

Testosterone appears to have a bone-preserving effect, but the cellular mechanism is not well understood. Studies have found a positive correlation between reduced testosterone levels and low bone mineral density (BMD), which can be reversed with testosterone supplementation.[13-15] As detailed above, testosterone is important for maintaining bone formation.[7]

TABLE 1. EFFECT OF SEX HORMONES ON BONE METABOLISM

Hormone	Effect
Estrogen	Suppress bone turnover Decrease osteoclast formation, activity, and lifespan Extend osteoblast lifespan Decrease bone response to PTH
Testosterone	Decrease bone resorption Increase osteoblast formation and lifespan Decrease osteoclast lifespan Promote periosteal apposition of the bone

Abbreviation: PTH, parathyroid hormone.

HYPOGONADISM IN THE CKD POPULATION

In addition to normal decreases in gonadal steroids that occur with aging and menopause, endocrine dysfunction leading to premature hypogonadism or impaired gonadal function is a common feature of CKD.[16]

Hypogonadism in women

Women with CKD experience menopause on average more than 4 years earlier than healthy women.[17] Females with CKD have lower estradiol peaks, lower follicle-stimulating hormone (FSH) to luteinizing hormone (LH) ratios, and higher prolactin levels. This suggests that early amenorrhea and anovulation may be due to a defect in the normal hypothalamic regulation of gonadotropin secretion.[18]

Possible effects of hypogonadism in women with CKD Stage 5 include sexual dysfunction, increased cardiovascular disease, cognitive deterioration, and osteoporosis.[19] Studies in young, nonuremic women have demonstrated lower bone mass in those with amenorrhea as compared to those who were regularly menstruating.[20;21] A recent study evaluating the relationship of estrogen deficiency to bone mass in young women (<50 years of age) on hemodialysis found amenorrheic women had lower estrogen levels, higher FSH levels, increased markers of bone resorption, and significantly lower trabecular BMD than regularly menstruating women.[22]

Hypogonadism in men

Impaired gonadal function, with low testosterone levels, is prevalent in men with CKD.[23] The low testosterone levels are accompanied by slight increases in LH and FSH. Primary gonadal dysfunction in men with CKD is thought to be a major contributor to reduced androgen synthesis, but the modest elevation in gonadotropins seen (in the face of low testosterone) supports a central abnormality of the hypothalamic pituitary axis as well. The etiology of these sex hormone abnormalities is not well understood. It is interesting that gonadal dysfunction is not affected by maintenance dialysis, but is almost completely normalized after kidney transplantation.[24] While studies suggest that testosterone is an important determinant of bone formation in healthy men in the absence of kidney disease,[6;7] the impact of testosterone deficiency on bone mass in kidney disease has not been addressed.

OSTEOPOROSIS IN THE CKD POPULATION

The applicability of the term osteoporosis in the CKD population has been questioned.[25] The World Health Organization criteria for the diagnosis of osteoporosis is based on the comparison of dual-energy X-ray absorptiometry (DXA) measurements of lumbar spine and femoral neck BMD with the average BMD of young adults at the time of peak bone mass, defined as a *T-score*.[26] These criteria were developed in women with postmenopausal osteoporosis, and provide sufficiently robust predictions of fracture risk in the absence of kidney disease in the general population (Table 2). However, as detailed below, fracture risk does not correlate well with DXA measures of BMD in patients with CKD.[27;28] It has been proposed that the BMD classification for CKD patients be simplified into two categories, "normal/high bone density" and "low bone density" according to Z-scores (bone mass adjusted for age, sex, and gender) rather than T-score (bone mass adjusted for peak bone mass).[25] Additional research is needed to confirm the validity of this classification system.

TABLE 2. WHO BONE DENSITY CLASSIFICATION

Classification	Definition	Risk
Normal	Bone density is no more then 1 SD below the young adult normal value (T score > -1.0)	Fracture risk is low
Osteopenia (low bone mass)	Bone density is 1 SD to 2.5 SDs below the young normal adult value (T score of -1.0 to -2.5)	Fracture risk is 4 times greater compared to normal BMD
Osteoporosis	Bone density >2.5 SDs below the young adult normal value (T score < -2.5)	Fracture risk is 8 times greater compared to normal BMD
Severe osteoporosis	Bone density >2.5 SDs below the young adult normal value and there have been one or more fragility fractures (T score < -2.5)	Fracture risk is 20 times greater compared to normal BMD

Adapted from Cunningham et al., Am J Kidney Dis 43:566-571, 2004.

Abbreviations: BMD, bone mineral density; SD, standard deviation; WHO, World Health Organization.

When evaluating the overall health and strength of bone, both the density and quality need to be considered. DXA is, by far, the most widely used technique for measuring bone mass. However, DXA is a projectional technique in which three-dimensional objects are analyzed as two-dimensional. Bone is presented as the combined sum of cortical and trabecular bone mineral content (BMC) within the projected bone area, concealing the distinct structural characteristics. DXA provides an estimate of BMC expressed as grams per the area in cm^2 of a defined anatomical region (e.g., individual vertebrae, whole body, or hip). This areal BMD (g/cm^2) is not a measure of volumetric BMD (g/cm^3) because it provides no information about the depth of bone. In contrast, quantitative computed tomography (QCT) measures volumetric BMD within cortical and trabecular bone. Bone quality is a reflection of normal turnover, architecture, damage accumulation (microfractures) and repair, and mineralization. Some components of bone architecture, such as cortical thickness, can be measured with QCT. However, a bone biopsy with histomorphometry is required to assess bone turnover and mineralization.

CKD patients have significant abnormalities in bone turnover, due to alterations in vitamin D and PTH metabolism that affect bone quality. These patients also experience the generalized loss of bone density that occurs with aging. Hypogonadism has a negative effect on both bone structure and turnover.[29;30] Therefore, uremic patients can have low bone density in combination with a wide variety of functional abnormalities, from extremely high-turnover lesions associated with hyperparathyroidism to greatly reduced bone remodeling as part of adynamic bone disease. The optimal treatment of these two abnormalities may vary significantly.

The various metabolic bone disorders can affect trabecular and cortical bone differently. Hyperparathyroidism and estrogen deficiency have similar negative effects on cortical bone density and thickness, but contrasting effects on trabecular bone turnover.[31] QCT measures in the tibia illustrate the distinct structural effects of estrogen deficiency, ROD or SHPT, and glucocorticoid therapy on trabecular and cortical bone (Table 3).[32] It is important to note that the ROD was associated with preserved trabecular density but decreased cortical density. These discrete effects would not be identified using DXA.

TABLE 3. EFFECT OF METABOLIC BONE DISEASE ON TRABECULAR AND CORTICAL BONE* (SD SCORES)[32]

	Dialysis	Amenorrhea	Glucocorticoid
N	10	17	37
Age (Years)	20-45	20-40	34 ±7
Trabecular	+0.05 SD	-1.5 SD	-0.39
Cortical	-2.19 SD	-0.8 SD	-0.06

* Assessed by peripheral quantitative computed tomography.
  Abbreviation: SD, standard deviation.

Although the term osteoporosis may have limited diagnostic meaning in CKD, consideration of the underlying pathophysiology in determining a treatment course is valuable. While the majority of women on dialysis are postmenopausal, and premature amenorrhea occurs frequently in women with CKD, the role of estrogen deficiency and postmenopausal bone loss as contributing factors in the development of ROD is generally given little consideration. The contribution of osteoporosis to ROD may be masked by the rapid progression of altered bone metabolism that occurs as CKD progresses. This is supported by the histomorphometric findings that the prevalence of osteoporosis in CKD Stage 3 and 4 populations is as high as 25%, but decreases in the CKD Stage 5 population, while changes attributed to SHPT increase.[33]

RELATIONSHIP BETWEEN BONE MINERALIZATION DEFECTS AND CARDIOVASCULAR DISEASE

The risk of cardiovascular disease in CKD patients appears to be far greater than that in the general population. Even in patients with moderate CKD, plasma creatinine levels are strong predictors of cardiovascular disease.[34]

There is accumulating evidence supporting a link between vascular and bone disease. The Framingham Heart Study suggested a relationship between the magnitude of bone loss and the progression of abdominal aortic calcification.[35] In dialysis patients with nondiabetic nephropathy, intimal-media carotid thickness correlated strongly with bone mineral density Z-scores in trabecular bone.[36]

Calcification of the vasculature seems to follow a similar process to that in bone with matrix vesicle formation and mineralization. Calcified atherosclerotic lesions have been found to contain many of the same regulatory factors previously identified for bone,[37] and some appear to have a comparable role in regulating mineralization in either bone or vasculature.[38;39]

Osteoprotegerin (OPG) is a cytokine in the tumor necrosis factor (TNF) receptor family that inhibits osteoclastogenesis. OPG-deficient mice have been found to have not only significant abnormalities of their skeletal system, but also to exhibit marked medial arterial calcification, suggesting that OPG may play a role in the association between osteoporosis and vascular calcification.[40;41] Several other bone cell-associated proteins, such as matrix Gla protein (MGP) and bone morphogenetic proteins (BMPs) are now under investigation for their potential role in moderating vascular calcification.[42;43] A recent study in rats has suggested that bisphosphonates can inhibit vascular calcification at similar doses used to inhibit bone resorption, providing additional support for a relationship between osteoporosis and vascular calcification.[44]

The relationship among bone disease, vascular calcification, and atherosclerosis in CKD is an emerging field of study that may provide novel classes of therapeutics to treat both bone and cardiovascular disease.

ASSESSMENT OF BONE MINERALIZATION IN CKD

Dual X-ray absorptiometry

The role of DXA in the diagnosis and treatment of ROD is unclear. DXA provides information on bone quantity (mineral content/density) but not bone quality, which is significantly altered by abnormalities in bone turnover seen in CKD. DXA does not provide information on bone turnover and correlates poorly with bone histology in CKD, so it is not helpful in classifying the form of ROD (e.g., low-turnover adynamic bone disease versus high-turnover osteitis fibrosa).

Findings on the correlation of BMD measurements with fracture risk in the CKD population are inconsistent. Several studies have demonstrated a positive correlation between BMD and fractures,[2;45] but there appears to be a poor correlation with fracture rates when bone density is measured by lumbar spine DXA. In Stage 5 CKD patients, BMD did not differ significantly between those patients with vertebral or fragility fractures compared to patients without fractures.[27;28] These conflicting findings may be related to the site and technique used. Spinal BMD measurement might be affected by aortic calcifications frequently observed in CKD patients. In addition, trabecular bone sclerosis can occur with SHPT, resulting in an increased vertebral BMD, despite disruption of structural integrity.[46] This is supported by the finding that, in CKD patients, BMD measurements of the cortical bone in the radius correlated better with fracture rates than lumbar spine BMD.[28] Measurement of BMD at the hip and radius may give better precision with fewer artifacts. Further studies in the CKD population are needed to determine the optimum sites for DXA measurement.

Quantitative computed tomography (QCT)

QCT has distinct advantages over DXA in evaluating bone structure. It provides a three-dimensional image that is not affected by surrounding structures. It allows accurate measurement of bone dimensions and distinguishes between cortical and trabecular bone. This is particularly advantageous with ROD, where hyperparathyroidism can lead to sclerotic thickening of trabecular bone with increased BMD but also to enhanced resorption of cortical bone with significant reductions in BMD. In contrast, low-turnover bone disorders typically result in reductions in trabecular BMD.[47] The ability of QCT to characterize disease effects on cortical and trabecular bone is illustrated in Table 3.

THERAPEUTIC CONSIDERATIONS

Although patients with kidney disease are at increased risk for early menopause and osteoporosis, few postmenopausal women are prescribed hormone replacement therapy (HRT). A population-based cohort study of HRT use in postmenopausal women with CKD Stage 5 reported the prevalence of HRT prescription was 10.8%, significantly less than in the general postmenopausal population.[48] The coexistence of ROD and the lack of prospective clinical trials make treatment recommendations for osteoporosis and hypogonadism in CKD difficult. The effect of kidney failure on the pharmacokinetics of therapeutic agents routinely used in the general population has not been well studied, plus the alterations in bone turnover that accompany CKD may have significant effects on the overall action of these agents on bone. Due to the lack of long-term evaluation, safety issues remain a concern with all of the potential therapeutic agents discussed below.

Hormone Therapy in CKD

Testosterone

Testosterone replacement among hypogonadal men in the general population has been shown to reduce bone remodeling and increase BMD.[49;50] However, the role of testosterone in treating bone disease in CKD has not been studied.

Estrogen

In the general population, postmenopausal estrogen replacement therapy has been shown to preserve bone mass and reduce the risk of osteoporosis.[51-53] These findings were supported in the CKD population by a recent 1-year study in a small cohort of premenopausal women with amenorrhea, showing a beneficial effect of transdermal estrogen therapy with cyclic norestisterone acetate.[54] Therapy induced regular menses, increased libido, increased plasma 17β-estradiol, and decreased prolactin in all treated women, compared to controls. The treated women demonstrated increased spine BMD measured by DXA, while the controls had progressive bone loss. The effect on cortical bone was not addressed. There are no long-term studies evaluating the efficacy and safety of estrogen replacement therapy in CKD. The pharmacokinetic profile of estrogen therapy may also be affected by reduced kidney function.[55]

Estrogen can be given alone, as estrogen with cyclic progesterone, or as continuous estrogen and progesterone. Long-term estrogen therapy alone, without progesterone, has been associated with an increased risk of endometrial carcinoma, so it should be avoided in women who have not had a hysterectomy.

The lack of long-term experience and clinical studies, along with the recent findings of the Women's Health Initiative (WHI) Study makes it difficult to make recommendations for estrogen therapy in CKD. The WHI study is a randomized, controlled trial evaluating estrogen plus progesterone treatment in normal, postmenopausal women. While preliminary observations showed a significant reduction in hip and vertebral fractures in the estrogen/progesterone treatment arm, they also noted an increased risk of breast cancer, pulmonary embolism, and coronary and cerebrovascular disease after long-term therapy.[56] Until there are more controlled trials in CKD on which to base recommendations for estrogen replacement, it may be better to consider some of the alternative therapies before hormone therapy is prescribed regularly for CKD patients.

Selective estrogen receptor modulators

Selective estrogen receptor modulators (SERMS) are agents that have the ability to selectively stimulate or inhibit the estrogen receptors of different target tissues. Raloxifene and tamoxifen are SERMS currently available for clinical use.

In a large study of women with osteoporosis and normal kidney function, raloxifene at a dose of 60 mg per day for 3 years increased lumbar spine BMD by 2.7% and decreased the incidence of vertebral fracture by 41%.[57] The rate of hip and other nonvertebral fractures was not affected. Plasma lipid values were also shown to decrease with raloxifene administration.[58]

The effect of raloxifene on bone metabolism and plasma lipid profile has been studied in postmenopausal women on dialysis.[59] In this double-blind controlled study, raloxifene (60 mg/day) was administered to women with documented osteoporosis. After one year of treatment, there was a significant increase in lumbar spine BMD that was accompanied by a decrease in bone resorption markers (plasma pyridinoline). Low-density lipoprotein (LDL) cholesterol levels decreased significantly without change in plasma triglycerides, total cholesterol, or high-density lipoprotein (HDL) cholesterol. No increase in side-effects was observed in the group treated with raloxifene.

Clinical trials in the general population and in dialysis patients have shown a promising effect of raloxifene on bone and lipid metabolism. However, the long-term effects of SERMS in CKD have yet to be evaluated.

Tibolone

Tibolone is a synthetic steroid whose metabolites have tissue-specific estrogenic, androgenic, and progestagenic actions. Tibolone has a long history of use in Europe, but has not yet been approved for use in the U.S. The beneficial effects of tibolone on BMD in postmenopausal women have been established.[60] It also appears to alleviate symptoms of menopause and improve sexual function, without the estrogenic effect on breast and endometrial tissue.

There have been no reported clinical trials with tibolone in the CKD population. One promising finding is the lack of effect of impaired kidney function on plasma levels of tibolone's active metabolites in a recent pharmacokinetic study.[61]

Bisphosphonates

Bisphosphonates are widely used in the general population and are effective in increasing BMD and decreasing fracture risk.[62] The use of bisphosphonates in CKD has not been adequately studied. While the kidney is a primary route of elimination for these drugs, they are removed efficiently by dialysis, such that the total clearance of bisphosphonates in hemodialysis patients is similar to that in healthy subjects.[63]

The potential long-term effect of bisphosphonate deposition in bone is of concern in CKD. These agents might be effectively used to reduce bone loss associated with high bone turnover in SHPT. While the amount of skeletal deposition of these drugs appears to be related to bone turnover, there is still significant bone uptake in dialysis patients with low bone turnover.[64] Therefore, indiscriminate use of bisphosphonates could lead to further suppression of bone turnover and increased potential for adynamic bone disease.

CONCLUSIONS

The role of hypogonadism and postmenopausal osteoporosis should not be overlooked when evaluating skeletal health in CKD patients. Clearly, additional controlled clinical trials in the CKD population are needed to determine the value of BMD measurements and the safety and efficacy of the various therapies to prevent bone loss. The decision to treat should be based on an evaluation of the benefits and risks for the individual patient, and should include collaboration (description and disclosure) with the patient.

REFERENCES

1. Alem AM, Sherrard DJ, Gillen DL, Weiss NS, Beresford SA, Heckbert SR, Wong C, Stehman-Breen C: Increased risk of hip fracture among patients with end-stage renal disease. Kidney Int 58:396-399, 2000

2. Atsumi K, Kushida K, Yamazaki K, Shimizu S, Ohmura A, Inoue T: Risk factors for vertebral fractures in renal osteodystrophy. Am J Kidney Dis 33:287-293, 1999

3. Coco M, Rush H: Increased incidence of hip fractures in dialysis patients with low serum parathyroid hormone. Am J Kidney Dis 36:1115-1121, 2000

4. Seeman E: Pathogenesis of bone fragility in women and men. Lancet 359:1841-1850, 2002

5. Riggs BL, Khosla S, Melton LJ, III: A unitary model for involutional osteoporosis: estrogen deficiency causes both type I and type II osteoporosis in postmenopausal women and contributes to bone loss in aging men. J Bone Miner Res 13:763-773, 1998

6. Slemenda CW, Longcope C, Zhou L, Hui SL, Peacock M, Johnston CC: Sex steroids and bone mass in older men. Positive associations with serum estrogens and negative associations with androgens. J Clin Invest 100:1755-1759, 1997

7. Falahati-Nini A, Riggs BL, Atkinson EJ, O'Fallon WM, Eastell R, Khosla S: Relative contributions of testosterone and estrogen in regulating bone resorption and formation in normal elderly men. J Clin Invest 106:1553-1560, 2000

8. Eriksen EF, Colvard DS, Berg NJ, Graham ML, Mann KG, Spelsberg TC, Riggs BL: Evidence of estrogen receptors in normal human osteoblast-like cells. Science 241:84-86, 1988

9. Horowitz MC: Cytokines and estrogen in bone: anti-osteoporotic effects. Science 260:626-627, 1993

10. Jilka RL, Hangoc G, Girasole G, Passeri G, Williams DC, Abrams JS, Boyce B, Broxmeyer H, Manolagas SC: Increased osteoclast development after estrogen loss: mediation by interleukin-6. Science 257:88-91, 1992

11. Naveh-Many T, Almogi G, Livni N, Silver J: Estrogen receptors and biologic response in rat parathyroid tissue and C cells. J Clin Invest 90:2434-2438, 1992

12. Reichel H, Koeffler HP, Norman AW: The role of the vitamin D endocrine system in health and disease. N Engl J Med 320:980-991, 1989

13. Karasek M, Kochanski JW, Bierowiec J, Suzin J, Swietoslawski J: Testosterone levels and bone mineral density in young healthy men and in young infertile patients. Neuroendocrinol Lett 21:25-29, 2000

14. Khosla S, Melton LJ, III, Atkinson EJ, O'Fallon WM, Klee GG, Riggs BL: Relationship of serum sex steroid levels and bone turnover markers with bone mineral density in men and women: a key role for bioavailable estrogen. J Clin Endocrinol Metab 83:2266-2274, 1998

15. Scane AC, Sutcliffe AM, Francis RM: Osteoporosis in men. Baillieres Clin Rheumatol 7:589-601, 1993

16. Palmer BF: Sexual dysfunction in uremia. J Am Soc Nephrol 10:1381-1388, 1999

17. Gipson D, Katz LA, Stehman-Breen C: Principles of dialysis: special issues in women. Semin Nephrol 19:140-147, 1999

18. Lim VS, Henriquez C, Sievertsen G, Frohman LA: Ovarian function in chronic renal failure: evidence suggesting hypothalamic anovulation. Ann Intern Med 93:21-27, 1980

*19. Weisinger JR, Bellorin-Font E: Outcomes associated with hypogonadism in women with chronic kidney disease. Adv Chronic Kidney Dis 11:361-370, 2004

20. Prior JC, Vigna YM, Schechter MT, Burgess AE: Spinal bone loss and ovulatory disturbances. N Engl J Med 323:1221-1227, 1990

21. Schachter M, Shoham Z: Amenorrhea during the reproductive years—is it safe? Fertil Steril 62:1-16, 1994

22. Weisinger JR, Gonzalez L, Alvarez H, Hernandez E, Carlini RG, Capriles F, Cervino M, Martinis R, Paz-Martinez V, Bellorin-Font E: Role of persistent amenorrhea in bone mineral metabolism of young hemodialyzed women. Kidney Int 58:331-335, 2000

23. Schmidt A, Luger A, Horl WH: Sexual hormone abnormalities in male patients with renal failure. Nephrol Dial Transplant 17:368-371, 2002

24. Prem AR, Punekar SV, Kalpana M, Kelkar AR, Acharya VN: Male reproductive function in uraemia: efficacy of haemodialysis and renal transplantation. Br J Urol 78:635-638, 1996

*25. Cunningham J, Sprague SM, Cannata-Andia J, Coco M, Cohen-Solal M, Fitzpatrick L, Goltzmann D, Lafage-Proust MH, Leonard M, Ott S, Rodriguez M, Stehman-Breen C, Stern P, Weisinger J: Osteoporosis in chronic kidney disease. Am J Kidney Dis 43:566-571, 2004

26. World Health Organization. Assessment of fracture risk and its application to screening for postmenopausal osteoporosis. Technical Report Series 843. 1994. Geneva, Switzerland.

Ref Type: Report

*27. Jamal SA, Chase C, Goh YI, Richardson R, Hawker GA: Bone density and heel ultrasound testing do not identify patients with dialysis-dependent renal failure who have had fractures. Am J Kidney Dis 39:843-849, 2002

28. Yamaguchi T, Kanno E, Tsubota J, Shiomi T, Nakai M, Hattori S: Retrospective study on the usefulness of radius and lumbar bone density in the separation of hemodialysis patients with fractures from those without fractures. Bone 19:549-555, 1996

29. Jackson JA, Kleerekoper M, Parfitt AM, Rao DS, Villanueva AR, Frame B: Bone histomorphometry in hypogonadal and eugonadal men with spinal osteoporosis. J Clin Endocrinol Metab 65:53-58, 1987

30. Riggs BL, Khosla S, Melton LJ, III: Sex steroids and the construction and conservation of the adult skeleton. Endocr Rev 23:279-302, 2002

31. Parfitt AM: A structural approach to renal bone disease. J Bone Miner Res 13:1213-1220, 1998

32. Tsurusaki K, Ito M, Hayashi K: Differential effects of menopause and metabolic disease on trabecular and cortical bone assessed by peripheral quantitative computed tomography (pQCT). Br J Radiol 73:14-22, 2000

33. Infante, M, Hernandez, G, Rojas, E, Fuenmayor N, Domínguez J, Suniaga O, Weisinger JR, and Bellorin-Font E. The spectrum of renal bone disease in chronic kidney disease (CKD) stages 3 to 5: Possible contribution of osteoporosis. J Am Soc Nephrol 14, 471A. 2003. Ref Type: Abstract

34. Shlipak MG, Simon JA, Grady D, Lin F, Wenger NK, Furberg CD: Renal insufficiency and cardiovascular events in postmenopausal women with coronary heart disease. J Am Coll Cardiol 38:705-711, 2001

35. Kiel DP, Kauppila LI, Cupples LA, Hannan MT, O'Donnell CJ, Wilson PW: Bone loss and the progression of abdominal aortic calcification over a 25 year period: the Framingham Heart Study. Calcif Tissue Int 68:271-276, 2001

*36. Nakashima A, Yorioka N, Tanji C, Asakimori Y, Ago R, Usui K, Shigemoto K, Harada S: Bone mineral density may be related to atherosclerosis in hemodialysis patients. Osteoporos Int 14:369-373, 2003

37. Tintut Y, Demer LL: Recent advances in multifactorial regulation of vascular calcification. Curr Opin Lipidol 12:555-560, 2001

38. Hofbauer LC, Schoppet M: Osteoprotegerin: a link between osteoporosis and arterial calcification? Lancet 358:257-259, 2001

39. Parhami F, Demer LL: Arterial calcification in face of osteoporosis in ageing: can we blame oxidized lipids? Curr Opin Lipidol 8:312-314, 1997

40. Bucay N, Sarosi I, Dunstan CR, Morony S, Tarpley J, Capparelli C, Scully S, Tan HL, Xu W, Lacey DL, Boyle WJ, Simonet WS: Osteoprotegerin-deficient mice develop early onset osteoporosis and arterial calcification. Genes Dev 12:1260-1268, 1998

41. Min H, Morony S, Sarosi I, Dunstan CR, Capparelli C, Scully S, Van G, Kaufman S, Kostenuik PJ, Lacey DL, Boyle WJ, Simonet WS: Osteoprotegerin reverses osteoporosis by inhibiting endosteal osteoclasts and prevents vascular calcification by blocking a process resembling osteoclastogenesis. J Exp Med 192:463-474, 2000

42. Bostrom KI: Cell differentiation in vascular calcification. Z Kardiol 89 Suppl 2:69-74, 2000

*43. Davies MR, Lund RJ, Hruska KA: BMP-7 is an efficacious treatment of vascular calcification in a murine model of atherosclerosis and chronic renal failure. J Am Soc Nephrol 14:1559-1567, 2003

44. Price PA, Faus SA, Williamson MK: Bisphosphonates alendronate and ibandronate inhibit artery calcification at doses comparable to those that inhibit bone resorption. Arterioscler Thromb Vasc Biol 21:817-824, 2001

45. Fontaine MA, Albert A, Dubois B, Saint-Remy A, Rorive G: Fracture and bone mineral density in hemodialysis patients. Clin Nephrol 54:218-226, 2000

46. Piraino B, Chen T, Cooperstein L, Segre G, Puschett J: Fractures and vertebral bone mineral density in patients with renal osteodystrophy. Clin Nephrol 30:57-62, 1988

47. Schober HC, Han ZH, Foldes AJ, Shih MS, Rao DS, Balena R, Parfitt AM: Mineralized bone loss at different sites in dialysis patients: implications for prevention. J Am Soc Nephrol

9:1225-1233, 1998

48. Stehman-Breen CO, Gillen D, Gipson D: Prescription of hormone replacement therapy in postmenopausal women with renal failure. Kidney Int 56:2243-2247, 1999

49. Behre HM, Kliesch S, Leifke E, Link TM, Nieschlag E: Long-term effect of testosterone therapy on bone mineral density in hypogonadal men. J Clin Endocrinol Metab 82:2386-2390, 1997

50. Katznelson L, Finkelstein JS, Schoenfeld DA, Rosenthal DI, Anderson EJ, Klibanski A: Increase in bone density and lean body mass during testosterone administration in men with acquired hypogonadism. J Clin Endocrinol Metab 81:4358-4365, 1996

51. Effects of hormone therapy on bone mineral density: results from the postmenopausal estrogen/progestin interventions (PEPI) trial. The Writing Group for the PEPI. JAMA 276:1389-1396, 1996

52. Ettinger B, Genant HK, Cann CE: Long-term estrogen replacement therapy prevents bone loss and fractures. Ann Intern Med 102:319-324, 1985

53. Studd J, Savvas M, Waston N, Garnett T, Fogelman I, Cooper D: The relationship between plasma estradiol and the increase in bone density in postmenopausal women after treatment with subcutaneous hormone implants. Am J Obstet Gynecol 163:1474-1479, 1990

54. Matuszkiewicz-Rowinska J, Skorzewska K, Radowicki S, Sokalski A, Przedlacki J, Niemczyk S, Wlodarczyk D, Puka J, Switalski M: The benefits of hormone replacement therapy in premenopausal women with oestrogen deficiency on haemodialysis. Nephrol Dial Transplant 14:1238-1243, 1999

55. Ginsburg ES, Owen WF, Jr., Greenberg LM, Shea BF, Lazarus JM, Walsh BW: Estrogen absorption and metabolism in postmenopausal women with end-stage renal disease. J Clin Endocrinol Metab 81:4414-4417, 1996

56. Rossouw JE, Anderson GL, Prentice RL, LaCroix AZ, Kooperberg C, Stefanick ML, Jackson RD, Beresford SA, Howard BV, Johnson KC, Kotchen JM, Ockene J: Risks and benefits of estrogen plus progestin in healthy postmenopausal women: principal results From the Women's Health Initiative randomized controlled trial. JAMA 288:321-333, 2002

57. Ettinger B, Black DM, Mitlak BH, Knickerbocker RK, Nickelsen T, Genant HK, Christiansen C, Delmas PD, Zanchetta JR, Stakkestad J, Gluer CC, Krueger K, Cohen FJ, Eckert S, Ensrud KE, Avioli LV, Lips P, Cummings SR: Reduction of vertebral fracture risk in postmenopausal women with osteoporosis treated with raloxifene: results from a 3-year randomized clinical trial. Multiple Outcomes of Raloxifene Evaluation (MORE) Investigators. JAMA 282:637-645, 1999

58. Barrett-Connor E, Grady D, Sashegyi A, Anderson PW, Cox DA, Hoszowski K, Rautaharju P, Harper KD: Raloxifene and cardiovascular events in osteoporotic postmenopausal women: four-year results from the MORE (Multiple Outcomes of Raloxifene Evaluation) randomized trial. JAMA 287:847-857, 2002

59. Hernandez E, Valera R, Alonzo E, Bajares-Lilue M, Carlini R, Capriles F, Martinis R, Bellorin-Font E, Weisinger JR: Effects of raloxifene on bone metabolism and serum lipids in postmenopausal women on chronic hemodialysis. Kidney Int 63:2269-2274, 2003

60. Modelska K, Cummings S: Tibolone for postmenopausal women: systematic review of randomized trials. J Clin Endocrinol Metab 87:16-23, 2002

61. Timmer CJ, Doorstam DP: Effect of renal impairment on the pharmacokinetics of a single oral dose of tibolone 2.5 mg in early postmenopausal women. Pharmacotherapy 22:148-153, 2002

62. Liberman UA, Weiss SR, Broll J, Minne HW, Quan H, Bell NH, Rodriguez-Portales J, Downs RW, Jr., Dequeker J, Favus M: Effect of oral alendronate on bone mineral density and the incidence of fractures in postmenopausal osteoporosis. The Alendronate Phase III Osteoporosis Treatment Study Group. N Engl J Med 333:1437-1443, 1995

63. Ala-Houhala I, Saha H, Liukko-Sipi S, Ylitalo P, Pasternack A: Pharmacokinetics of clodronate in haemodialysis patients. Nephrol Dial Transplant 14:699-705, 1999

64. Saha H, Ala-Houhala I, Ylitalo P, Kleimola T, Pasternack A: Skeletal deposition of clodronate is related to parathyroid function and bone turnover in dialysis patients. Clin Nephrol 58:47-53, 2002

*Suggested Reading

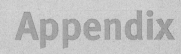

Appendix

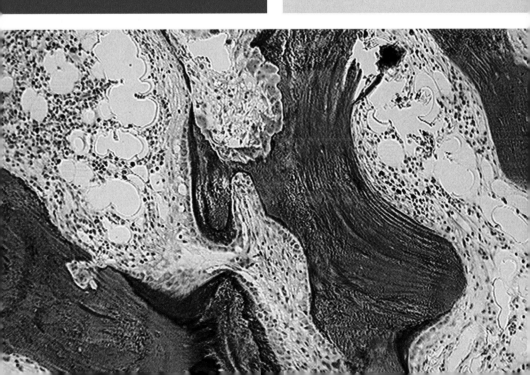

TABLE 1. CONVERSION FACTORS OF METRIC UNITS TO SI UNITS

Test	Metric Unit	Conversion Factor	SI Unit
Calcium	mg/dL	0.25	mmol/L
Calcium ionized (plasma)	mg/dL	0.25	mmol/L
Phosphorus (plasma)	mg/dL	0.323	mmol/L
Magnesium (plasma)	mg/dL	0.41	mmol/L
Creatinine (plasma)	mg/dL	83.30	μmol/L
Blood urea nitrogen (plasma)	mg/dL	0.36	mmol/L
Albumin (plasma)	g/dL	10.00	g/L
Alkaline phosphatase (plasma)	IU/L	0.02	μkat/L
Intact parathyroid hormone (plasma)	pg/mL	0.105	pmol/L
25(OH)$_2$D (serum or plasma)	ng/mL	2.5	nmol/L
1.25(OH)$_2$D (serum or plasma)	pg/mL	2.4	pmol/L

Note: Metric Units x Conversion Factor = SI Units
SI Units/Conversion Factor = Metric Units

TABLE 2. CLASSIFICATION OF CHRONIC KIDNEY DISEASE (CKD)

CKD Stage	GFR Range (mL/min/1.73m^2)	Description
1	≥90	Kidney damage with normal or elevated GFR
2	60-89	Kidney damage with slightly lowered GFR
3	30-59	Moderately lowered GFR
4	15-29	Severly lowered GFR
5	<15	Kidney failure

Note: In this guide, the term CKD is used as a general term for CKD Stages 3-5, as this is when manifestations of bone and mineral metabolism become apparent.

Adapted from: Levey et al., Kidney Intl 67:2089-2100, 2005

Abbreviations: CKD, chronic kidney disease; GFR, glomerular filtration rate

TABLE 3. TARGET LEVELS FOR PTH, CALCIUM, AND PHOSPHORUS BY STAGE OF CKD

CKD Stage	GFR Range (mL/min/1.73m^2)	Intact PTH (pg/mL)	Total Corrected Plasma Calcium (mg/dL)	Plasma Phosphorus (mg/dL)	CaXP (mg^2/dL^2)
3	≥30-59	35-70 pg/mL (3.85-7.7 pmol/L)	Normal range for laboratory	2.7-4.6 (0.87 mL-1.49 mmol/L)	<55
4	15-29	70-110 pg/mL (7.7-12.1 pmol/L)	Normal range for laboratory	2.7-4.6 (0.87 mL-1.49 mmol/L)	<55
5	<15	150-300 pg/mL (16.5-33 pmol/L)	8.4-9.5 (2.10-2.37 mmol/L)	3.5-5.5 (1.13-1.78 mmol/L)	<55

Based on K/DOQI Clinical Practice Guidelines for Bone Metabolism and Disease in CKD, Am J Kidney Dis 42:1-201, 2003.

Abbreviations: CKD, chronic kidney disease; GFR, glomerular filtration rate; PTH, parathyroid hormone.

TABLE 4. CALCIUM CONTENT OF COMMON CALCIUM-BASED PHOSPHATE BINDERS

Compound	Brand Name	Compound Content (mg)	Elemental Calcium (mg)	# of pills to provide 1,500 mg elemental calcium*
Calcium Acetate	Phoslo®	667	167	9
Calcium Carbonate	Chooz™ (Gum) TUMS™ (Regular)	500 mg	200 mg	7.5
	TUMS EX™	750 mg	300 mg	5
	TUMS Ultra™	1,000 mg	400 mg	3.75
	LiquiCal	1,200 mg	480 mg	3
	CalciChew™ CalciMix™ Oscal 500™ TUMS 500™	1,250 mg	500 mg	3
	Caltrate 600™ NephroCalci™	1,500 mg	600 mg	2.5
Calcium Citrate	Citra-Cal®			Not Recommended
Calcium Acetate/ Magnesium Carbonate	MagneBind® 200	450 Ca acetate/ 200 Mg Carb	113 (Mg = 57)	13
	MagneBind®	300 Ca acetate/ 300 Mg Carb	76 (Mg = 85)	20

*Maximum recommended daily calcium intake from K/DOQI Clinical Practice Guidelines for Bone Metabolism and Disease in CKD. Am J Kidney Dis 42:1-201, 2003.

TABLE 5. SUMMARY OF CLINICALLY USEFUL PHOSPHATE BINDERS

Phosphate Binder	Common Product Name	Advantages	Potential Side Effects/Disadvantages
Aluminum-based	Aluminum Hydroxides: Amphojel® Alu-Caps® Alu-Tabs® AltenaGEL® Dialume® Aluminum Carbonate: Basojel® Carafate®	High phosphate binding capacity Does not add to calcium load Inexpensive Readily accessible	High potential for aluminum toxicity and bone mineral defects with long term use Constipation GI Distress Chalky taste
Calcium carbonate	Tums® Oscal® Calcichew® Caltrate® Calci-mix® Titralac® Chooz gum®	Inexpensive Readily accessible	Hypercalcemia Extraskeletal calcification Constipation
Calcium acetate	PhosLo®	Higher phosphate binding capacity and less calcium absorption than calcium carbonate	Hypercalcemia Extraskeletal calcification Constipation
Magnesium-based	MagneBind® (Magnesium carbonate and calcium carbonate combination)	Less total calcium load	Diarrhea, Potential for magnesium toxicity Potential for hyperkalemia.
Sevelamer	RenaGel®	Does not add to calcium load Demonstrated to reduce the risk of cardiovascular calcification Reduces cholesterol levels	Requires large doses/pill size which may effect patient compliance Decreases bicarbonate possibly enhancing metabolic acidosis. Potentially effects absorption of lipid soluble vitamins GI Distress Expensive
Lanthanum	Fosrenal®	Does not add to calcium load	Potential for accumulation of lanthanum in bone

TABLE 7. ABBREVIATIONS AND ACRONYMS

β_2M	β_2-microglobulin
β_2MA	$\beta_2$2-microglobulin amyloidosis
ABD	Adynamic bone disease
ADHR	Autosomal dominant hypophosphatemic rickets
AP	Alkaline phosphatase
Arb2	Adrenergic receptor 2
AVN	Avascular necrosis
BMC	Bone mineral content
BMD	Bone mineral density
BMP	Bone morphogenetic protein
BSAP	Bone-specific alkaline phosphatase
CAPD	Continuous ambulatory peritoneal dialysis
CaSR	Calcium-sensing receptor
CaXP	Calcium-phosphorus product
CKD	Chronic kidney disease
CRP	C-reactive protein
CsA	Cyclosporine
CT	Computed tomography
CUA	Calcific uremic arteriolopathy
CV	Cardiovascular
DBP	Vitamin D-binding protein
DFO	Deferoxamine
DM	Diabetes mellitus
DOPPS	Dialysis Outcomes and Practice Patterns Study
DPD	Deoxypyridinoline
DRA	Dialysis-related amyloidosis
DXA	Dual-energy x-ray absorptiometry
EBCT	Electron-beam computed tomography
ECaC	Epithelial calcium channel
ECaR	Extracellular calcium-sensing receptors
ECG	Electrocardiogram
FGF	Fibroblast growth factor

FSH . . . . Follicle-stimulating hormone

GBMI . . . . Global Bone and Mineral Initiative

GH, rhGH . . . . Growth hormone, recombinant human growth hormone

HDL . . . . High-density lipoprotein

ICTP . . . . Procollagen Type 1 cross-linked carboxy-terminal telopeptide

IGF . . . . Insulin-like growth factor

IL . . . . Interleukin

KDIGO . . . . Kidney Disease: Improving Global Outcomes

K/DOQI . . . . Kidney Disease Outcomes Quality Initiative

LDL . . . . Low-density lipoprotein

LH . . . . Luteinizing hormone

MGP . . . . Matrix gla protein

MRI . . . . Magnetic resonance imaging

MSCT . . . . Multislice (spiral) computed tomography

NCX . . . . Calcium exchanger

OM . . . . Osteomalacia

OPG . . . . Osteoprotegerin

PICP . . . . Procollagen type 1 carboxy-terminal extension peptides

PTG . . . . Parathyroid gland

PTH, iPTH . . . . Parathyroid hormoneintact parathyroid hormone

PTHrP . . . . Parathyroid hormone-related peptide

PTX . . . . Parathyroidectomy

PWV . . . . Pulse wave velocity

PYD . . . . Pyridinoline

QCTqCT . . . . Quantitative computed tomography

RANKL . . . . Receptor activator of NF-κB ligand

RIA . . . . Radioimmunoassay

ROD . . . . Renal osteodystrophy

RR . . . . Relative risk

SD . . . . Standard deviation

SDS . . . . Standard deviation scores

SERMS . . . . Selective estrogen receptor modulators

SHPT . . . . Secondary hyperparathyroidism

TGFβ	Transforming growth factor-β
TIO	Tumor-induced osteomalacia
TNF	Tumor necrosis factor
USRDS	United States Renal Data System
VC	Vascular calcification
VDR	Vitamin D receptor
VSMC	Vascular smooth muscle cell
WHI	Women's Health Initiative
XLH	X-linked hypophosphatemic rickets